Economic Consequences of Noncommunicable Diseases and Injuries in the Russian Federation

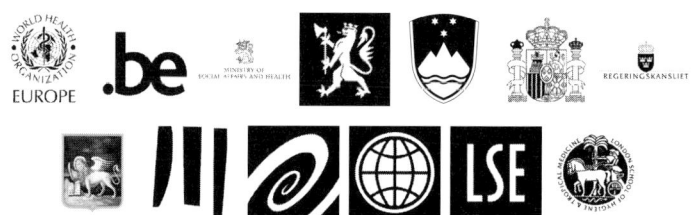

The European Observatory on Health Systems and Policies supports and promotes evidence-based health policy-making through comprehensive and rigorous analysis of health systems in Europe. It brings together a wide range of policy-makers, academics and practitioners to analyse trends in health reform, drawing on experience from across Europe to illuminate policy issues.

The European Observatory on Health Systems and Policies is a partnership between the World Health Organization Regional Office for Europe, the Governments of Belgium, Finland, Norway, Slovenia, Spain and Sweden, the Veneto Region of Italy, the European Investment Bank, the Open Society Institute, the World Bank, the London School of Economics and Political Science and the London School of Hygiene & Tropical Medicine.

Economic Consequences of Noncommunicable Diseases and Injuries in the Russian Federation

Marc Suhrcke, Lorenzo Rocco, Martin McKee,
Stefano Mazzuco, Dieter Urban and Alfred Steinherr

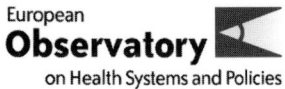

European
Observatory
on Health Systems and Policies

Keywords:
CHRONIC DISEASE – economics
WOUNDS AND INJURIES – economics
COST OF ILLNESS
RUSSIAN FEDERATION

Please address requests about the publication to: Publications, WHO Regional Office for Europe, Scherfigsvej 8, DK-2100 Copenhagen Ø, Denmark

Alternatively, complete an online request form for documentation, health information, or for permission to quote or translate, on the Regional Office web site (http://www.euro.who.int/PubRequest)

The views expressed by authors or editors do not necessarily represent the decisions or the stated policies of the European Observatory on Health Systems and Policies or any of its partners.

The designations employed and the presentation of the material in this publication do not imply the expression of any opinion whatsoever on the part of the European Observatory on Health Systems and Policies or any of its partners concerning the legal status of any country, territory, city or area or of its authorities, or concerning the delimitation of its frontiers or boundaries. Where the designation "country or area" appears in the headings of tables, it covers countries, territories, cities, or areas. Dotted lines on maps represent approximate border lines for which there may not yet be full agreement.

The mention of specific companies or of certain manufacturers' products does not imply that they are endorsed or recommended by the European Observatory on Health Systems and Policies in preference to others of a similar nature that are not mentioned. Errors and omissions excepted, the names of proprietary products are distinguished by initial capital letters.

The European Observatory on Health Systems and Policies does not warrant that the information contained in this publication is complete and correct and shall not be liable for any damages incurred as a result of its use.

ISBN 9 789289 021906

Printed in the United Kingdom by The Cromwell Press, Trowbridge, Wilts.

Contents

List of tables, figures and boxes

Tables

Figures

Boxes

About the authors

Martin McKee is Professor of European Public Health at the London School of Hygiene & Tropical Medicine (LSHTM), where he co-directs the School's European Centre on Health of Societies in Transition, and he is also a research director at the European Observatory on Health Systems and Policies. His main fields of research include health systems, the determinants of disease in populations, and health policy, all with a focus on eastern Europe and the former Soviet Union.

Stefano Mazzuco, PhD, is Research Assistant in the Department of Statistical Sciences at the University of Padova. He obtained a PhD from the University of Padova in 2003. His main current research interests are demographic economics, with special reference to poverty and family formation and transition to adulthood.

Lorenzo Rocco, PhD, is Assistant Professor of Economics with the University of Padova in Italy. He obtained a PhD from the University of Toulouse I in 2005. His main current fields of research are development economics and health economics.

Alfred Steinherr is Head of the Department of Macro-Analysis and Forecasting at the German Institute for Economic Research (DIW Berlin), Professor of Economics at the Free University of Bolzano, executive in residence and professor at the Sacred Heart University Luxembourg, and with the European Investment Bank, Luxembourg. His main current fields of research include business cycle forecasting, labour economics, and financial markets.

Marc Suhrcke, PhD, is an economist with the WHO Regional Office for Europe in Venice, Italy, where he is in charge of the Health and Economic Development workstream. His main current research interests are the economic consequences of health, the economics of prevention and the socio-economic determinants of health.

Dieter Urban, PhD, is Assistant Professor for Economics at Johannes Gutenberg University in Mainz, Germany. He obtained his PhD from Copenhagen Business School and previously held research positions at the London School of Economics and Bocconi University. He teaches panel data econometrics to graduate students. In his research, he undertakes macro- and microeconometric studies in many fields of economics, including health economics. He is also an affiliate of CESifo in Munich.

Acknowledgements

The work on this report was undertaken in large part as input into the World Bank report *Dying too young: addressing premature mortality and ill-health due to noncommunicable diseases and injuries in the Russian Federation*, published in 2005.

The World Bank's support for the contribution of Lorenzo Rocco and for two consultative visits to Moscow by Marc Suhrcke and one by Martin McKee is gratefully acknowledged. We have particularly appreciated the very active support and encouragement of Patricio Marquez (World Bank). Charles Griffin, Cem Mete, Edmundo Murrugara, Willy De Geyndt, Christoph Kurowski, Derek Yach and John Litwack provided very useful and extensive comments on a previous draft. Many thanks go to Elizabeth Goodrich and Nicole Satterley for copy-editing the text. Many of the results presented are the direct output of parallel work coordinated and undertaken by Marc Suhrcke, Lorenzo Rocco, and Martin McKee on a forthcoming report on health and economic development in eastern Europe and central Asia. Dieter Urban, Stefano Mazzuco, and Alfred Steinherr made key contributions to the present report. Financial support for the contribution of the latter three co-authors has been provided by the WHO European Office for Investment for Health and Development in Venice, Italy. Thanks also to Andrea Bertola for support on a number of data issues and Theadora Koller (both WHO Venice Office) for editorial advice. We are also grateful to Giovanna Ceroni from the European Observatory for managing the publication process.

All remaining errors are the sole responsibility of the authors. Views expressed here are exclusively the authors' and do not necessarily correspond to the official views of their affiliated organizations.

Executive summary

There is increasing evidence of the two-way relationship between health and economic growth. While economic development can lead to improved population health, a more healthy population can also drive economic growth. Similarly, at the level of the individual, while greater wealth contributes to better health, good health is an important determinant of economic productivity. This finding has important policy implications: national and international policy-makers interested in promoting the economic development of a country should seriously consider the role health investment could play in achieving their economic policy goals. Yet little is known about the direct relevance of these recent findings for the transition countries in central and eastern Europe and the Commonwealth of Independent States (CIS) that are facing a very particular health challenge, predominantly comprising noncommunicable diseases (NCD) and injuries. To date, their economic implications have hardly been analysed. This study takes a first step towards analysing the issue. The focus is the Russian Federation, although the findings are also relevant to other transition economies. In particular, we begin to answer two important questions.

- What effect has adult ill-health, in particular NCD and injuries, had on the Russian economy and the economic outcomes of the people living there?

- If the excessive burden of adult ill-health in the Russian Federation were reduced, what economic benefits could result?

The overarching message from our findings is unambiguous: poor adult health negatively affects economic well-being at the individual and household levels in the Russian Federation; and, if effective action were taken, improved health would play an important role in sustaining high economic growth rates.

Our findings relating to the first question are as follows.

- A simple, conservative estimate indicates significant costs of absenteeism due to illness.

- Ill-health appears to have had a significant and sizeable impact on labour productivity in recent years, but less so on labour supply.

- However, the labour supply has been significantly and sizeably affected to the extent that jobholders suffering from chronic illness have retired as a result.

- Severe alcohol consumption significantly increases the probability of losing one's job.

- The death of a household member affects surviving household members' welfare and behaviour in at least two ways, i.e. by increasing the probability of depression and of increased alcohol consumption.

- Chronic illness has negatively affected household incomes, particularly during the period 1998–2002.

The second part of this study assesses the macroeconomic benefits that would accrue by reducing NCD and injury mortality rates among adults in the Russian Federation. The main conclusion is that these benefits would be substantial for the Russian economy, irrespective of how they are evaluated. This occurs despite the fact that we assess only the effect of mortality reductions, setting aside morbidity reduction, which would probably attend mortality improvement and almost certainly also be sizeable. Our main findings are set out here.

- The static economic benefit (i.e. valuing a life year gained by one gross domestic product (GDP) per capita) of gradually bringing the Russian Federation's adult NCD and injury mortality rates down to the most recent rates for European Union (EU) Member States (those belonging to the EU prior to May 2004) by 2025 is estimated to be between 3.6% and 4.8% of the 2002 Russian GDP.

- The broadly defined "welfare" benefits (i.e. using a "value of life" measure) from achieving the rates of the EU Member States (those belonging to the EU prior to May 2004) by 2025 are estimated to be as high as 29% of the 2002 Russian GDP.

- The dynamic benefits (i.e. the effect on economic growth rates) are massive and growing over time. Even if the future returns are discounted to the starting-year value (2002), they represent a multiple of the static GDP effects.

The third part of the study briefly examines the potential response to the findings obtained, identifying some of the institutional barriers to effective action and setting out some of the policy options.

We have not directly taken into account the costs of different health interventions, the next logical step towards a full economic assessment, but the expected economic benefits would easily exceed any reasonable increase in investments to maintain and promote health, both inside and outside the health system. Another logical step will be to assess the benefits that would accrue from the morbidity reductions expected from those same investments.

These findings have obvious implications for economic and health policy-makers in the Russian Federation as well as for international organizations interested in the country's social and economic development: investing in the health of the Russian adult population should be seriously considered as one (of several) means by which to achieve economic policy goals. Furthermore, while the analyses were possible in the Russian Federation because of the existence of appropriate data, it is likely that similar findings would be obtained from other economies in transition, given the similarity of their health and economic situations. Hopefully, this report will be a stimulus to other countries in the region to reassess the priorities they place on investment in health as one of the drivers of economic growth.

Chapter 1

Introduction

There is increasing evidence of the two-way relationship between health and economic growth. While economic development can lead to improved population health, a more healthy population can also drive economic growth.[1] This has important policy implications: national and international policy-makers interested in promoting the economic development of a country should seriously consider the role that health investment could play to further the achievement of their economic policy goals.

Little is known about the relevance of these recent findings for the Russian Federation. Yet it is difficult to believe that the Russian economy and the individuals disproportionately hit by ill-health would not face a severe economic penalty. The Russian Federation is one of very few countries where life expectancy has been decreasing in recent years (McMichael et al. 2004), and the Russian Federation's health status compares very unfavourably with those of its economic competitors.

Direct evidence that actually measures the impact of poor health on the Russian economy, or, by extension, the gains that might be achieved by reducing avoidable disability and premature death, is scant. One exception is a study (Ladnaia, Pokrovsky and Rühl 2003) that estimates the impact of different scenarios for progression of the HIV/AIDS epidemic on the Russian Federation's macroeconomic prospects. The authors quantify the prohibitive price that the Russian Federation would pay, in foregone economic growth, if the HIV/AIDS epidemic were left unchecked. Yet while HIV/AIDS is an

---

[1] This case was made cogently in the 2001 report of the Commission on Macroeconomics and Health (CMH 2001) for the developing country context, and more recently, the evidence on the economic benefits of health for high-income countries was assembled in Suhrcke et al. (2005).

extremely serious threat to both the health and economy of the Russian Federation, the predominant share of the *current* disease and mortality burden involves NCD and injuries. Shkolnikov, McKee and Leon (2001) report that it is not only the historically low level of life expectancy but also the recent reduction in life expectancy that have been driven by mortality from cardiovascular disease (CVD) and injuries. It is also apparent that much of the premature mortality in the Russian Federation occurs disproportionately at ages between 40 and 55, normally a person's most productive years.

What, then, is the effect of ill-health among adults in the Russian Federation, in particular that due to NCD and injuries, on both the Russian economy and the economic prospects of individual Russians and their families? And what would be the economic benefits of reducing the very high burden of disability and premature mortality among Russian citizens?

This report provides an overview of a series of newly undertaken studies of the economic consequences of health in the Russian Federation, conducted within the framework of a World Bank-led study of the Russian mortality crisis (World Bank 2005). To the best of our knowledge, this is the first comprehensive effort to provide empirical evidence on the economic consequences of adult ill-health in the Russian Federation. We focus on NCDs and injuries, which, according to the World Bank (2005), account for most of the Russian Federation's ill-health. While there is clearly room for further work on this subject, the message from these analyses is unambiguous: the poor adult health of Russians negatively affects economic well-being at the individual and household levels, and improving adult health can be expected to contribute significantly to sustained economic growth.

In presenting our results on the impact of health on the economy, we are also aware that the relationship between health and economic growth works both ways. It is explicitly not our purpose to argue that the contribution of health to the economy is more important than the contribution of the economy to health. Whether one is more important than the other is debatable and is in any case unnecessary to ask. Here, it is sufficient to show that there is certainly a path from health to the economy. It is this mutually reinforcing relationship between health and the economy that provides a higher return from investing a given amount of resources in both, compared with investing the same amount in either.

Although based on data from the Russian Federation, the findings from these analyses also contribute to our understanding of the economic implications of NCD and injuries in other countries. There is comparatively little research on this subject, in particular in relation to low- and middle-income countries.

The relative lack of a convincing economic argument for investing in policies that will combat NCD and injuries may help to explain why these conditions have had so little attention from policy-makers (Yach and Hawkes 2004).

This study is structured as follows. In Chapter 2, we briefly sketch a conceptual framework that highlights some of the channels through which health determines economic outcomes. Chapter 3 presents the key epidemiological facts about adult health in the Russian Federation. Some of these facts already provide highly suggestive evidence of the potential economic importance of adult (ill-)health in the Russian Federation. Chapter 4 presents the core of this study: the empirical evidence on the micro- and macroeconomic impact of health in the Russian Federation. Chapter 5 examines a potential response to the findings obtained, identifying barriers to effective action and setting out some policy options. Chapter 6 presents our convictions derived from the findings presented in the earlier chapters.

Chapter 2

Conceptual framework

Figure 2.1 shows the channels through which health could contribute to an economy and ultimately to economic growth. Four channels are shown, though others may exist: enhanced labour productivity, higher labour supply, higher skills from better education and training, and more savings available for investment in physical and intellectual capital. Figure 2.1 also illustrates that as an economy develops, health improves.

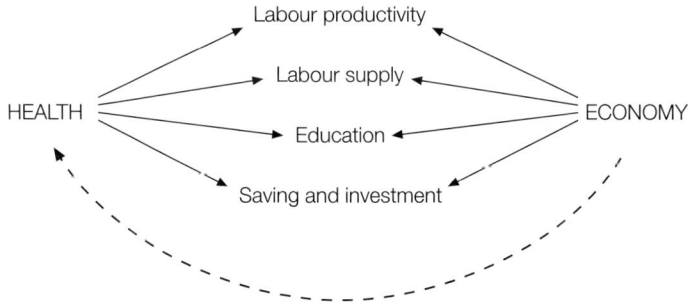

Figure 2.1 *From health to wealth (and back)*
Source: Modified from Bloom, Canning and Jamison 2004.

Labour productivity

Healthier individuals could reasonably be expected to produce more per hour worked. First, productivity would be increased directly by enhanced physical and mental activity. Second, more physically and mentally active individuals would make better and more efficient use of technology, machinery, and equipment. A healthier labour force could also be expected to be more flexible and adaptable to changes (e.g. in job tasks and the organization of labour), reducing job turnover with its associated costs (Currie and Madrian 1999).

Labour supply

Somewhat counter-intuitively, economic theory predicts a more ambiguous impact of health on labour supply. The ambiguity results from two effects that offset each other. The first effect – the *substitution* effect – suggests that as lower productivity from poor health leads to reduced wages, workers will respond to the lower returns by working less. Thus, as more leisure is pursued, the labour supply is constricted. The second effect – the *income* effect – suggests that as poor health leads to reduced wages, workers will work more to recoup lost income, thus expanding the labour supply. The income effect is likely to gain importance if the social benefit system fails to cushion the effect of reduced productivity on lifetime earnings. The net impact of the substitution and income effects thereby ultimately becomes an empirical question (Currie and Madrian 1999).

Education

Human capital theory suggests that more educated individuals are more productive (and obtain higher earnings). Accepting that children with better health and nutrition achieve higher education attainments and suffer less from school absenteeism or dropping out of school early, improved health in early years would contribute to raising future productivity. Moreover, if good health is also linked to higher life expectancy, healthier individuals would have more incentive to invest in education and training, as the rate of depreciation of the gains in skills would be lower (Strauss and Thomas 1998).

Saving and investment

The health of an individual or a population is likely to have an impact not only on the level of income but also on the distribution of income among savings, consumption, and investment. Individuals in good health are likely to have a wider time horizon, so their savings ratio may be higher than that of individuals in poor health. Therefore, a population experiencing a rapid increase in life expectancy may, other things being equal, be expected to have higher savings. This should also result in a higher propensity to invest in physical or intellectual capital (Bloom, Canning and Graham 2003).

Chapter 3
Adult ill-health in the Russian Federation

The Russian Federation is one of only a few countries where life expectancy is falling. However, the situation in the Russian Federation and its ex-Soviet neighbours differs from some other countries where life expectancy is also falling, such as in sub-Saharan Africa, where the declines have been driven by the HIV/AIDS epidemic. In the former, both the recent declines and the current low level of life expectancy were driven largely by increasing mortality among people of working age, with the greatest contribution from NCD and injuries (Shkolnikov et al. 2004; Nolte, McKee and Gilmore 2005). As a consequence, the global development agenda, driven by the pursuit of the Millennium Development Goals (MDGs), may not be perfectly appropriate for the Russian case (and for most other eastern European countries). A recent World Bank report showed how reducing mortality from CVD and injury would have a much greater impact on life expectancy than achieving the health-related MDGs (child and maternal mortality, reductions in HIV/AIDS and tuberculosis (TB)) (Lock et al. 2002; Rechel, Shapo and McKee 2004).

The scale of the challenge is apparent from Table 3.1, which shows that although male life expectancy at birth in the Russian Federation is about two years less than in Brazil or Poland, the probability that a 15-year-old Russian boy will die before he reaches 60 is over 40%, about 16 percentage points higher than in Brazil, double the rate of Turkey, and quadruple that of the United Kingdom.

The fact that a major determinant of a population's health is its country's level of economic development may in part explain some of the differences in mortality rates depicted in Table 3.1. However, as Figure 3.1 shows, even if we take income differences into account, Russian male mortality rates are still

Table 3.1 *Life expectancy and adult mortality in selected countries*

Country	Life expectancy at birth (years) total (2001)	Probability of dying between ages 15 and 60 (% males) (2000 to 2001)	Probability of dying between ages 15 and 60 (% females) (2000 to 2001)
Russian Federation	**66**	**42.4**	**15.3**
Japan	81	9.8	4.4
France	79	13.7	5.7
United States	78	14.1	8.2
Germany	78	12.6	6.0
United Kingdom	77	10.9	6.6
Denmark	77	12.9	8.1
Mexico	73	18.0	10.1
Poland	70	22.8	8.8
Turkey	70	21.8	12.0
Brazil	68	25.9	13.6
Kyrgyzstan	66	33.5	29.9

Source: World Bank 2003.

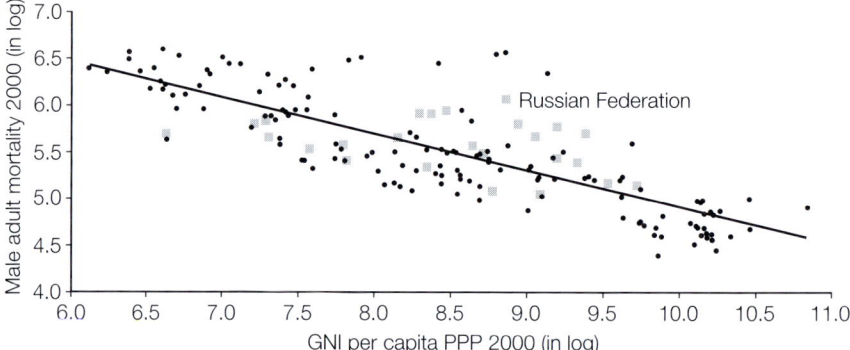

Figure 3.1 *Male adult mortality and gross national income (GNI) per capita in 2000*

Note: Squares indicate countries in eastern Europe and central Asia. PPP: purchasing power parity
Source: World Bank 2004.

substantially higher than those of other countries with a similar level of per-capita income. The only countries that are on a still higher trajectory than the Russian Federation are those that have suffered some of the worst HIV/AIDS crises (e.g. Botswana, South Africa, Namibia, Swaziland).

The social consequences of this high toll of avoidable mortality are bound to be significant. The widely held view that NCDs exclusively strike people that have passed retirement age is mistaken. In the Russian Federation the young and the middle-aged are by far more affected than in western Europe. Figure 3.2 illustrates this point by displaying the ratio of mortality in the Russian Federation from CVD in different age groups to that in Sweden. While the death rate is between two and three times higher in older ages, it is a remarkable 12 times higher in the 30–34 age group. A similar, slightly less acute difference is seen for deaths from injuries (Figure 3.3).

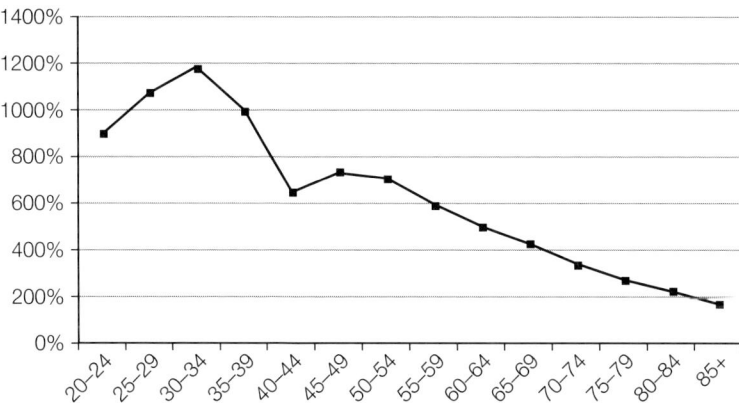

Figure 3.2 *Cardiovascular mortality rates in the Russian Federation as a percentage of those of Sweden*
Source: WHO Regional Office for Europe 2006.

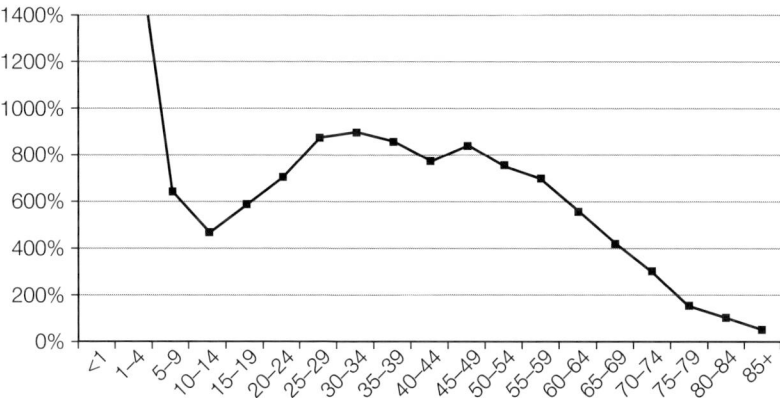

Figure 3.3 *Injury mortality rates in the Russian Federation as a percentage of those of Sweden*
Source: WHO Regional Office for Europe 2006.

The difference between the Russian Federation and western Europe is even greater when their morbidity rates are compared (Table 3.2). An analysis of healthy life expectancy – i.e. life expectancy augmented by a morbidity component – demonstrates the less well-recognized phenomenon of a high level of ill-health among women, in particular those of working age. Indeed, the difference in healthy life expectancy between the Russian Federation and western Europe is even higher than that for life expectancy alone. This confirms that morbidity data contain important information not captured by mortality/life expectancy data. If the Russian health crisis is not merely a health crisis of men, as these findings very strongly suggest, then the economic costs of ill-health are most likely also felt among women.

Table 3.2 *Life expectancy and healthy life expectancy in the Russian Federation*

	Country/Region	At age 20		At age 40		At age 65	
		LE	*HLE*	*LE*	*HLE*	*LE*	*HLE*
Males	Russian Federation	41.9	36.7	22.4	17.3	11.4	6.7
	Western Europe	54.5	50.4	31.2	27.6	15.0	12.5
Females	Russian Federation	54.2	40.6	31.1	18.5	15.2	5.8
	Western Europe	60.2	53.7	36.0	30.3	18.1	14.0
Female–male gap (years)	Russian Federation	12.3	3.9	8.7	1.2	3.9	-0.9
	Western Europe	5.7	3.3	4.8	2.7	3.1	1.5

Notes: HLE (healthy life expectancy) is calculated by Sullivan's method (Sullivan 1971); LE: life expectancy.
Source: Andreev, McKee and Shkolnikov 2003.

In sum, this chapter shows that the health challenges facing the Russian Federation affect not only the retired, but also working-age people – and very much so. Moreover, in contrast to what mortality data alone tell us, women's health has been seriously affected, too. This purely epidemiological evidence alone would suggest that ill-health during middle age has a substantial impact on economic outcomes at the individual and aggregate levels. Chapter 4 examines this issue in depth.

Empirical evidence on the economic impact of health in the Russian Federation

This chapter presents a selection of empirical evidence on various channels through which health has contributed or might contribute to a number of economic outcomes in the Russian Federation. Section 4.1 focuses specifically on the assessment of the economic impact of ill-health in the Russian Federation in recent years. Most of our evidence in this chapter is microeconomic, as this is the level of analysis that most readily allows assessment of the economic impact of ill-health.[2] Section 4.2 looks forward by estimating the likely future economic benefits that could be reaped from improving adult health in the Russian Federation in three plausible scenarios.

4.1 What has been the impact of adult (ill-)health on economic outcomes?

After assessing the impact of adult health on economic status in the Russian Federation, our main findings are as follows:

- A simple, conservative estimate indicates significant costs of absenteeism due to illness.

- Ill-health appears to have had a significant and sizeable impact on labour productivity in recent years, but less so on labour supply, at least among jobholders.

---

[2] We have not undertaken a macroeconomic assessment of the impact of health on the past macroeconomic performance since the onset of transition in the early 1990s, because we believe that it would be very hard to detect such a causal impact of health in this very transitional period. Nor do we focus on the role of health in determining economic outcomes in the pre-transition period. This has been carried out, for instance, by Davis (2005). He shows that there is much to suggest that the early post-Second World War health achievements made in the former Soviet Union contributed significantly to the comparatively strong economic development in the period up to the early 1970s. However, these health achievements were made in the area of communicable diseases and child and maternal health, not in NCDs and injuries.

- However, the labour supply has been significantly and sizeably affected to the extent that jobholders suffering from chronic illness have retired as a result of such illness.

- Severe alcohol consumption significantly increases the probability of losing one's job.

- The death of a household member affects surviving household members' welfare and behaviour in at least two ways, i.e. by increasing the probability of depression and increased alcohol consumption.

- Chronic illness has negatively affected household incomes, particularly during the period 1998–2002.

Since the most visible economic impact of adult ill-health runs via the labour market, we pay most attention to this mechanism (Subsection 4.1.1). Subsequently, we briefly explore the broader impact of chronic illness health on income (Subsection 4.1.2) and the effect of adult mortality on the remaining household members (Subsection 4.1.3).

4.1.1 The impact of health on labour market outcomes

We attempt here to assess various ways in which (ill-)health has had an impact on the labour market in the Russian Federation. It appears intuitively obvious that an individual's health status has an impact on *labour supply* – i.e. the number of hours worked and the decision whether to participate in the labour force – as well as on *labour productivity* – the output produced per unit of time worked (commonly proxied by the hourly or daily wage rate). However, what seems obvious is not always the outcome of scientific reasoning and research. As explained in Chapter 2, economic theory predicts an unequivocally negative impact of ill-health on labour productivity, but an ambiguous one on labour supply.

In what follows we summarize our results on the impact of ill-health on labour supply and productivity in the Russian Federation. In particular, we present estimates of the impact of health status on labour supply and productivity, using two different datasets: the Russian Longitudinal Monitoring Survey and the NOBUS Household Survey (the Appendix has descriptions of the datasets). Moreover, we propose an estimate of the effects of chronic illness on early retirement (as one dimension of labour supply) based on data from the Russian Longitudinal Monitoring Survey (RLMS) and, by slightly changing the perspective, the effects of alcohol on the probability of being fired. This is followed by an attempt to estimate the impact of adult mortality on surviving household members in terms of probability of subsequent alcohol consumption and depression. Finally, we produce a longitudinal analysis of the effect of health problems on income.

4.1.1.1 The cost of work absenteeism due to illness

On average 10 days are lost per employee per year due to illness in the Russian Federation, while the average for Member States belonging to the EU prior to May 2004 is just below 8 days. Work absenteeism due to illness is a widely used, if imperfect, illustration of the effect of illness on the labour supply of individuals. In the 15 Member States belonging to the EU prior to May 2004, for instance, a survey conducted in 2000 found that on average 17% of workers reported having been absent from work at least once in the previous 12 months due to health problems (European Foundation for the Improvement of Living and Working Conditions 2001). These absences represent an average loss of 7.9 working days per worker. Sickness absence incurs the direct cost of the sickness benefits paid to absent employees (when applicable) as well as the indirect cost of lost productivity during the time away from work. In the United Kingdom in 1994, lost productivity due to sickness absence was assessed at over £11 billion (€15.8 billion). In Portugal, 5.5% of all working days in the 2000 largest enterprises were assessed to have been lost in 1993 as a result of illness and accidents. In Belgium, €2.8 billion was paid in 1995 in sickness benefits and benefits for work-related injuries and occupational diseases. In 1993, payments to cover work absence were assessed to be up to €30.6 billion in Germany and €15.8 billion in the Netherlands (€3.9 billion for benefits for sickness absence and €11.9 billion for disability benefits) (see European Foundation for the Improvement of Living and Working Conditions (1997) for data on costs of absenteeism). Figure 4.1 shows the annual average number of work days missed due to illness in the Russian Federation (2000) – calculated using data from the RLMS – compared with the latest available figures for the 15 Member States belonging to the EU prior to May 2004. Although this indicator has a disadvantage in that it reflects both the burden of ill-health and the incentives created by the employment policy environment, it does serve as a useful illustrative example.

The overall cost associated with the reported work days lost due to illness in the Russian Federation varies between 0.55% and 1.37% of GDP, depending on the estimation method (Table 4.1). The monthly absenteeism figures from Figure 4.1 can be converted to a monetary value either by using the average wage rate (resulting in the lower value: column 1) or the GDP per capita (resulting in the higher value: column 3) (details of the calculations are in given in Table A.1 in the Appendix). This is a significant impact, given that the indicator fails

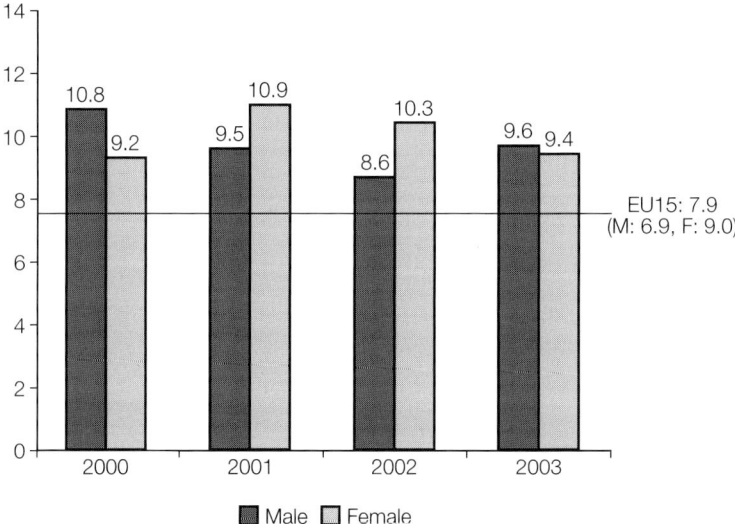

Figure 4.1 *Annual average days of absence due to illness per employee in the Russian Federation (2000–2003) and EU Member States before May 2004 (2000)*
Notes: The Russian figures are obtained by multiplying the monthly RLMS figures by 12; EU15: Member States belonging to the EU before 1 May 2004.
Sources: Russian Federation data are from RLMS rounds 9–12. EU15 data refer to the year 2000 and are from the European Survey of Working and Living Conditions, 2000.

Table 4.1 *Costs of absenteeism due to illness in the Russian Federation*

	Total wage loss (US$ billion)	Total wage loss as % of GDP	Total production (GDP) loss (US$ billion)	Total production loss as % of GDP
2000	40.33	0.55%	97.38	1.34%
2001	52.01	0.68%	105.17	1.37%
2002	56.62	0.71%	104.03	1.30%
2003	60.96	0.71%	112.87	1.31%

Note: The annual average missed days in the Russian Federation are obtained by multiplying the RLMS monthly figures by 12. For details of the calculations see the Appendix.
Source: Calculations based on RLMS absenteeism data.

to capture the many other ways in which ill-health has an impact on the labour market. In particular, it does not take into account the effect of the reduction of productivity, nor does it capture the impact on mortality. In a theoretical model, Pauly et al. (2002) examine the magnitude and incidence of costs associated with absenteeism under a range of assumptions (size of the firm, the production function, the nature of the firm's product, and the competitiveness of the labour market). They conclude that the cost of lost work time can be substantially higher than the wage when perfect substitutes are not available to replace absent workers, when production involves teamwork, or where a penalty is associated with failing to meet an output target.

Absenteeism as such is a somewhat crude indicator of the effect of ill-health on the labour market, as is this valuation method, which neglects many other ways in which ill-health has an impact on the labour market. Nor does this method claim to demonstrate a causal relationship. The following subsections use more structural analyses.

4.1.1.2 The impact of health on labour supply and labour productivity

This subsection examines the impact of ill-health on the labour supply and on labour productivity among jobholders in the Russian Federation. (There are a number of methodological challenges involved in properly analysing the issue. Box 4.1 and the Appendix provide technical details.) We also explore the role of health in determining participation in the labour market.

Significant research[3] has explored the labour market impact of ill-health in high-income countries. This research demonstrates a negative impact of ill-health both on labour productivity and on labour supply. Mitchell and Burkhauser (1990) used the United States Survey of Disability and Work in 1978 to find that arthritis reduced wages by 27.7% for men and 42.0% for women. Moreover, it reduced the number of hours worked by 42.1% and 36.7% respectively, for men and women. Stern (1996), using the United States Panel Study on Income Dynamics of 1981, showed that limited ability to work due to illness reduced wages by 11.7% and 23.8% for men and women, respectively, when a selection correction for participation in the labour force was introduced. In addition, the probability of staying outside the labour force increased by an estimated 13%. Using the same data, Haveman et al. (1994) estimated that (lagged) ill-health decreased worked hours by 7.4%. Berkovec and Stern (1991), using data from the National Longitudinal Survey of Older Men (1966–1983), found that poor health status reduced wages by 16.7%. Baldwin, Zeager and Flacco (1994), using data from the Survey of Income and Program Participation of 1984, found that health limits reduced wages by 6.1% for men and 5.4% for women. While the varying percentages from these studies lead to theoretical ambiguity, at least in high-income countries there is overall more evidence of a significant negative impact of ill-health on labour supply than on productivity (i.e. wage rates).

Among jobholders, ill-health appears to have had a significant and sizeable impact on labour productivity – but less so on labour supply – in the Russian Federation in recent years. The impact also seems to be more pronounced among males than females. These findings, while slightly different from some in Organisation for Economic Co-operation and Development (OECD) countries, are not necessarily surprising, since the social welfare system in the

---

[3] For an extensive review see, for example, Currie and Madrian (1999) and Suhrcke et al. (2005).

Russian Federation operates very differently than those in OECD countries, affecting the relationship between health and the labour market. In fact, the finding of a significant impact on the wage rate rather than on hours worked is evidence of health's particularly strong economic impact. (Subsection 4.1.1.3 presents evidence of the existence of one labour supply effect of, in particular, chronic illness and its impact on early retirement.)

The fact that the results obtained using the different methods are qualitatively similar tends to confirm the validity of our findings. We used various methods to develop a sufficiently robust and reliable picture of the labour market impact of adult health. Each method has its own way of addressing the methodological challenges involved in the analysis. In choosing the different approaches we have been guided by relevant literature. Details of our methodology and results are in Box 4.1.

Box 4.1 *Technical details and results of the impact of ill-health on labour supply and productivity*

Choosing methodologies is largely determined by data availability and by the informed evaluation of the importance of the endogeneity problem, which tends to afflict many, if not all, efforts to establish a causal relationship in economic and social empirical research. In the context of this study the endogeneity problem means that there could be a simultaneous relationship between the chosen health proxy and labour market outcomes that would bias the statistical relationship that would be measured using the most standard econometric technique (i.e. ordinary least squares estimation). The proposed solutions to the endogeneity problem also critically depend on the health indicator used and the potential measurement error associated with the given health indicator, because in some cases the particular kind of measurement error can offset the bias resulting from the endogeneity problem.

We have used three methods, all adopted from the existing literature. The main data source to which we applied the methods is the RLMS, specifically the four years from 1999 to 2002. We have also applied the second method (instrumental variable estimation) to the NOBUS household survey, which has been carried out only once: in 2003. As health proxy, we used a self-rated health indicator, medically diagnosed diseases, or work days missed owing to illness.

1. Ordinary least squares (OLS) regressions

This approach is based on a seminal paper by Bartel and Taubman (1979) that uses a Mincerian wage equation by adding to the usual variables (age, work experience, years of schooling, family background) some indicators of diseases, both physical and mental (heart disease and hypertension, psychoses and neuroses, arthritis, bronchitis, ulcers, diseases of the nerves, diseases of the liver and bone diseases). In particular, Bartel and Taubman analyse the effects of such diseases on the basis of their year of onset in order to disentangle short-term from long-term effects. We performed a similar exercise by regressing wage rates (in natural logarithms and at 2000 prices) and the number of hours worked per week (in natural logarithms) on a large set of the individual-specific health and non-health variables and environmental variables (Table A.2 in the Appendix lists these variables). The assumption in this approach – corroborated by a number of statistical tests – is that endogeneity does not really matter given the specific health indicators used, justifying the use of OLS.

Table A.3 and Table A.4 in the Appendix report the results of four models, respectively, that differ by date of medical diagnosis for diabetes, heart attack, stroke, TB and hepatitis (our dataset has data for only these diseases). We find that, as expected, lung, kidney and spine chronic diseases reduce the wage rate (and hence productivity). Surprisingly, chronic lung disease increases labour supply. Recently diagnosed heart attacks and TB reduce wage rate, as expected. Hepatitis diagnosed very early reduces labour supply while recently diagnosed TB increases it. Indeed, respiratory and lung-related diseases (such as asthma and bronchitis) seem to have a positive effect on labour supply. Given the fact that respiratory diseases cause relatively little limitation on work, a possible hypothesis explaining this puzzle could be that individuals seek to increase their revenue to compensate for their additional medical care costs.

Although this approach has been used in the literature, its underlying assumptions are controversial. The next two methods address endogeneity more directly.

2. Instrumental variables (IV) estimation

When endogeneity is explicitly taken into account, a "simultaneous equation" or "instrumental variables" approach is typically the preferred option. Following this method, the endogenous variable (here, the health indicator) should be substituted by the predicted values coming from its own regression over a set of instrumental variables plus all the exogenous variables that are part of the model. The researcher must choose as instruments one or more variables that are correlated with the endogenous variable but uncorrelated with the error term. The predicted values will then contain part of the information from the original variable, but they will be purified from the correlation with errors. This approach was applied to both the RLMS and the NOBUS data. Since the surveys differ, the precise specification of the estimation methodology also differs slightly.

➤➤

Box 4.1 *(cont.)*

RLMS

We used individual self-reported health status as the health proxy in the first set of regressions and the reported number of work days missed due to illness in the second. The latter is also self-reported, so it may be affected by measurement errors that are also systematically related to the individuals' characteristics. We used this indicator because it could be a more specific indicator of work limitations than the overall health status. Schultz and Tansel (1995) used the same indicator in another national context, interpreting it as an "objective" measure of health status. We have performed two kinds of estimations and both follow Stern (1989) in the choice of instruments. Stern used medically diagnosed diseases to instrument for self-reported health indicators.

The variables in the third column of Table A.2 in the Appendix are used as instruments for respectively self-evaluated health status and missed days due to ill-health (the chosen date of diagnosis for the last five is between 5 and 10 years before the interview).

Table A.5 and Table A.6 report estimates for both the logarithm of wage rate and labour supply, separately by gender. Both health indicators negatively affect the wage rate, but they do not have a significant influence on labour supply. *Reported good health status increases the wage rate by 22% for women and by 18% for men, compared to those who were not in good health. Similarly, a work day missed due to illness reduces the wage rate by 3.7% in the male subsample and by 5.5% among females.*

The Sargan test of overidentification (Sargan 1958) does not reject the hypothesis of exogeneity of the selected instruments. Although this result must be interpreted only as an indication of exogeneity, because the Sargan test has only little power, it does support the Bartel and Taubman (1979) assumption of exogeneity of the health conditions they used in their OLS analysis.

NOBUS

We used the NOBUS[4] survey exclusively for the instrumental variable procedure, and we again used the self-reported health status as a health proxy: the dummy *healthGOOD* comprises both "excellent" and "good" self-rated health status (as in the RLMS analysis). We used a two-stage least squares (2SLS) regression of the logarithm

---

[4] While the RLMS has certain advantages – in particular that it is repeated annually, allowing comparisons over time – the NOBUS survey, so far only held once (in 2003), covers a far larger share of the population – about 44 500 households – and is representative both nationally and for 46 of the larger subjects of the Russian Federation. It captures a range of aspects of household welfare and has a strong focus on household access to social services. Its health component is, however, very small compared to that in the RLMS and hence a direct comparison with the results from the RLMS reported above is not possible.

of monthly wage rate and the logarithm of worked hours per week respectively on age, gender, number of children, private sector employment, secondary school and university, length of work experience, location indicators and urban/rural indicator. Secondary school and university are represented by the values 2 and 3 of the categorical variable schooling derived from a NOBUS categorical variable that is ordered in 8 levels. Work experience length comes directly from a NOBUS categorical variable ordered in 5 levels. The urban indicator assumes value 1 for all places with more than 20 000 inhabitants. We included one location indicator for each region.

Individual health status was instrumented by the parents' health status. This may be justified because many chronic diseases are transmitted intergenerationally – either biologically or socially. Therefore, parents' health can be correlated with the health of their offspring without necessarily being correlated with the children's individual-specific omitted variables absorbed by the error term. This choice, determined by data availability, meant that we had to limit our analysis to the subsample of jobholders who lived in households with their parents. Clearly, this might cause a selection bias, which is not easy to address.

The results in Table A.7 and Table A.8 in the Appendix show that health has an impact on wages more than labour supply (among individuals who participate into the labour force). In particular, *males in good health earn about 30% more than others (i.e. males with fair, bad and very bad health), and females earn 18% more.*

The Sargan tests reported at the bottom of Table A.7 and Table A.8 generally support our choice of instruments (especially for females). We have tried other instruments, such as location indicators or the number of inhabitants to capture differences in the prevalence of communicable diseases, differences in the availability of medical facilities, differences in the prices of health inputs, and differences in environmental conditions. All these instruments were rejected by the Sargan test. Also, including parents' age in addition to parents' health status increased the probability of instruments' endogeneity.

Despite the positive signal previously offered by the Sargan test, concerns remain about the actual exogeneity of the chosen instruments. For instance, it seems reasonable to think that high levels of labour supply may increase the probability of stomach diseases and hypertension, because of the prolonged stress. Moreover, one may think that heart attacks, strokes or chronic heart diseases are linked to possible individual risky lifestyles (smoking, drinking, little physical exercise), which may be correlated with individual-specific error components. To address these concerns, we have moved from cross-sectional to panel analysis in the next approach.

▶▶

Box 4.1 *(cont.)*

3. Panel regressions

In this third approach we exploited the longitudinal dimension of the dataset by using panel regression methods. Few studies on the relationship between health and labour market outcomes have explicitly adopted panel data estimators. Recently, Pelkowski and Berger (2004) studied the impact of health on employment, wages and hours worked, distinguishing between temporary and permanent impairments by using fixed effects estimators. Here, we have followed another recent study, which makes extensive use of panel data analysis (Cotoyannis and Rice 2001). The authors suggest the use of Hausman-Taylor (HT) estimators (Hausman and Taylor 1981). In terms of our previous problem of finding "good" instruments, the main advantage of this procedure is that it does not require finding valid instruments outside the model, because it uses the already-included exogenous variables to instrument the relevant endogenous variable. The only requirement is the inclusion of both time-varying and time-invariant variables, each of which has to be separated into exogenous and endogenous ones. Moreover, HT estimators have the advantage over the usual within (fixed effects) estimators of allowing the effects of time-invariant variables to be consistently estimated. The disadvantage lies in the strong exogeneity assumptions to ensure consistency. For this reason, as in Cotoyannis and Rice (2001), we test such exogeneity assumptions by means of a (Hausman 1978) test. Moreover, to further improve the precision of our estimates, we also apply the Amemiya and Macurdy (AM) (1986) estimators, which share the same spirit as HT, but make use of a more efficient set of instruments (essentially transformations of the HT instruments). A Hausman test between HT and AM estimators favoured the latter.

To perform our study, we employed the sample of all individuals who have been followed in rounds 9–12 and who provided answers to all the questions in the survey we used. This means we can only consider the subsample of jobholders. Owing to attrition and the relatively high frequency of missing responses, the subsample of males has only 274 individuals, each observed four times, while the subsample of females has 476 individuals. To address the problem of an eventual selection bias, we performed similar estimations, whenever possible, on a significantly larger unbalanced panel, which, to our comfort, produced similar results.

The results are in Tables A.9–A.12 in the Appendix. In general, we found that *good health status increases wage rate for males, while it does not substantially affect labour supply. This result is in line with what is obtained in the cross-sectional instrumental variables estimators of the preceding subsection. However, now the effect of good health is reduced: being in good health increases the wage rate by about 7.5%. Surprisingly, good health does not have an impact either on wage rate or labour*

▶▶

supply among female workers, unlike what is seen in the cross-sectional instrumental variables estimations, where the effect on females was even greater than the effect on male wage rate.

For the sake of completeness, we used an alternative measure of health status: the "missed days due to ill-health" variable. However, its coefficient was statistically insignificant both in the wage rate and in the labour supply model.

4.1.1.3 The impact of chronic illness on early retirement

This subsection looks at a very specific potential labour supply effect of health: that of chronic illness on the decision to exit the labour force, to retire. It complements the preceding analysis that also partly looked at labour supply.

Many studies in industrialized countries have shown that ill-health, and in particular chronic illness, affects the decision to exit the labour force: healthy people, other things being equal, tend to retire later than less-healthy ones. Based on a review of various United States studies, Sammartino (1987) concluded that those in poor health are likely to retire between one and three years earlier than those in good health with similar economic and demographic characteristics. Bound, Stinebrickner and Waidmann (2003), based on the analysis of data from the American Health and Retirement Study, estimated that a representative individual in poor health is 10 times more likely than a similar person in average health to retire before becoming eligible for pension benefits. Coile (2003) found that health shocks have a large effect on labour supply decisions by both men and women, mainly when accompanied by major changes in functional status. For example, the onset of a heart attack or stroke accompanied by an important deterioration in the ability to perform "activities of daily living" (e.g. dressing) was estimated to reduce the number of work hours supplied by men per year by 1030 or to raise the probability of leaving the labour force by 42%. A comparable effect of a 654-hour decrease or a 31% increase in the probability of leaving the labour force was found for women.

Turning to evidence from European countries, Jiménez-Martin, Labeaga and Martínez (1999) found that health,[5] particularly among men, was a very relevant factor in the decision to retire and for their spouse to retire with them. The authors use information on labour market transitions between 1994 and 1995 from the European Community Household Panel, pooling data from

---

[5] The health variables generally refer to the year 1994 (to minimize the endogeneity bias) and include the following indicators: self-reporting good health, self-reporting a chronic physical or mental health problem (data available only for 1995), having been admitted as an inpatient during the previous year, having visited a doctor between one and five times in the year, and having visited a doctor more than five times in the year.

across the EU, to analyse retirement patterns of individuals and couples in a sample of men older than 54 years and women older than 49. Strong evidence of the influence of health status in the retirement decision is also found by Siddiqui (1997), using data from the German Socioeconomic Panel looking at men in western Germany who had reached the minimum retirement age (which, given the related policies in the country, is considered to be 58 years).[6] Indeed, the degree of disability seems to be the dominant factor explaining early retirement, with the probability of leaving the labour force at the earliest possible age for disabled men being four times that of men without disability. As Siddiqui notes, these results suggest that improving employees' health could be a highly effective measure to raise the actual age of retirement.

Applying the various approaches used in other countries to the Russian Federation's case reveals a statistically very robust and sizeable impact of chronic illness on both age of retirement and on the probability of retiring in the subsequent year. We followed two different, complementary approaches: a Cox regression and a panel logit regression. Controlling for other relevant determinants of the decision to retire (e.g. age, gender, income), both approaches confirm the finding that chronic illness increases the probability of retiring. The former approach (Cox regression) assesses the effect of chronic illness on the probability that an individual will retire in a given year after the first year of employment. This methodology's limitation is that we cannot be entirely sure about the direction of the causality – does ill-health predict retirement or vice versa? The second approach (the panel logit regression) is more appropriate to address this issue, since it examines the effect of chronic illness on the probability of retiring in the subsequent year.

The Cox regression indicates that a hypothetical male aged 55 on median income and having certain other characteristics[7] would be expected to retire at age 59, while a chronic illness would lower his expected retirement age by two years (Figure 4.2). While the technical details of the regression results (see Box 4.2) can be difficult to interpret, they are more intuitively understandable if applied to a hypothetical individual. Similar results are obtained for females. Strictly speaking, though, we can only talk about evidence of an *association* between chronic illness and earlier retirement, since the available data offer no way of discovering the time of onset of a chronic disease for an individual. In particular, we do not know whether the illness occurred before or after retirement, so we cannot say, from this analysis, whether the statistical association reflects the effect of chronic illness on retirement or vice versa. We can, however, address this issue by using a panel logit regression.

---

[6] The self-employed are withdrawn from the sample due to their different pension systems.
[7] The other characteristics are: married, has one child, not smoking, not drinking, of normal weight, with a high-school diploma, born in the Russian Federation and living in an urban area.

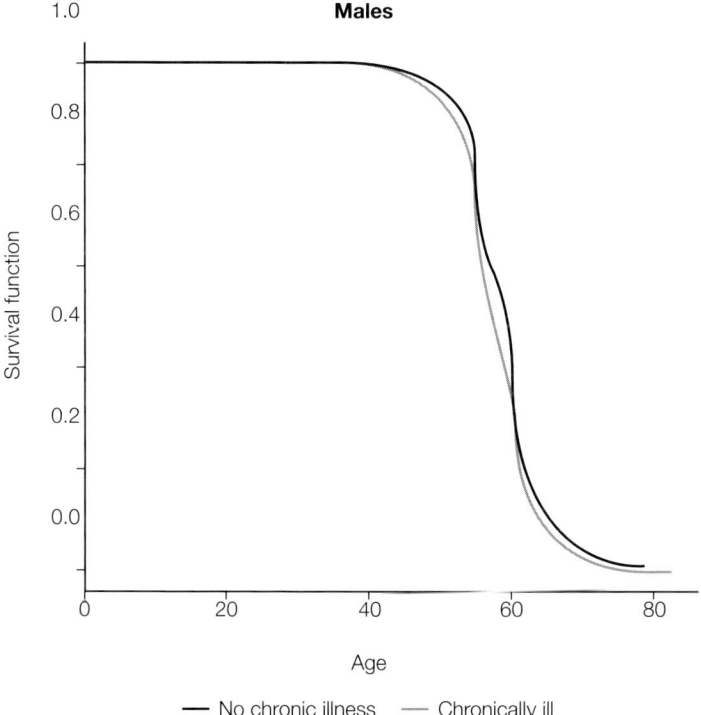

Figure 4.2 *Probability of remaining in the workforce with and without chronic illness, by age, based on Cox regression model*

Note: Cox regression results are described in Box 4.2
Source: Calculations based on RLMS round 11.

Box 4.2 *Cox regression: technical details and results*

A Cox regression allows us to estimate the precise moment that an event takes place as time proceeds. It is usually employed In survival analysis, where the outcome considered is death. It can also serve the purpose of estimating the timing of retirement. We estimated a Cox regression model on the age at retirement, using data from the 11th round of the RLMS (2002), where we can find retrospective information on job retirement.

Estimating a Cox regression model on the age at retirement: this is a model of a hazard regression where the log hazard function of retirement $\log[h(t)]$ is assumed to be a linear function of a baseline hazard function and the effect of p covariates. Formally:

$$\log[h(t)] = \log[h_0(t)] + \beta_1 x_1 + \beta_2 x_2 + \ldots + \beta_p x_p$$

Thus, the parameters we estimated represent a proportional shift of the baseline hazard function due to the covariates. A positive parameter means an increase in the risk of retiring from work during the overall time period (since first employment). The results are in Table 4.2. The reported coefficients should be interpreted as follows: a

Box 4.2 *(cont.)*

Table 4.2 *Results of Cox regression model on age to retirement*

Variable	Coefficient
Age	-.492***
Age squared	.003***
Female	-.423***
Age* female	.0132***
Married	-.275***
Cohabit	-.129
Widowed or divorced	-.262***
Chronic illness	.228***
Poverty status	.495***
Household income	-.0116***
Hh income* chronic illness	-.014**
High-school diploma	-.447***
No. of children < 7 years	-.123
Female* no. of children under 7	.378***
Born in Russian Federation	-.141***
Living in village	.113**

Notes: *** 1% significance level; ** 5% significance level; * 10% significance level; "Hh": Household head.

positive coefficient means an *increase* in the risk of experiencing the event (retirement from work in this case) and a negative coefficient is associated with a decrease in the risk of experiencing the event. (The test based on Schoenfeld residuals showed that the null hypothesis – the effect of chronic illness on the decision to retire being proportional – is not rejected.)

We controlled for a set of demographic and socioeconomic indicators: age, gender, income, education, etc. The health variable of particular interest is the presence of a chronic illness. A positive coefficient on the chronic illness variable indicates an increase in the probability (i.e. the hazard) of entering retirement, relative to the baseline first year of employment.

Those who are married, widowed or divorced are more likely to retire later from the job market than those who never married. The effect of age is U-shaped. Females retire later but the effect is weak and decreases with age. Smoking increases the risk of retiring, but the effect decreases with age. The effect of weight is interesting: those who are below the normal weight (in terms of body mass index) retire earlier, whereas those who are overweight or obese are more likely to retire later than individuals of normal weight. Reported drinking does not have any significant effect, but chronic illness has a positive and highly significant effect. This means that, after having controlled for other factors, we find that, in contrast with findings from the Kaplan-Meier estimates, those suffering from any chronic disease are more likely to retire earlier from the job market. Moreover, the effect of chronic illness interacts with income: the higher the income level the weaker the effect of chronic illness. In addition, we find that workers below the poverty line retire earlier and that income has a negative effect (i.e. the higher the income level, the later a worker retires). The number of children has no significant effect for males but it has a positive one for females. Finally, the estimates from the Cox model suggest that people born in the Russian Federation are more likely to retire than those born outside the Russian Federation, and those living in a village are more likely to retire earlier than those living in urban areas.

Table 4.3 *Random effects logit regression results*

Variable	Coefficient
Age	-0.492 ***
Age squared	0.003 ***
Reference: male	
Female	-0.423 ***
Age* female	0.013 ***
Married	-0.275 ***
Cohabit	-0.129
Widow or divorced	-0.262 ***
Chronic illness	**0.228** ***
Poverty status	0.495 ***
Household income	-0.012 ***
Income* chronic illness	**-0.014** **
High-school diploma	-0.447 ***
Number of children in household	-0.123
Female* no. of children	0.378 ***
Born in Russian Federation	-0.141 ***
Living in village	0.113 **
Constant	4.192 ***
Rho	0.141 **

Notes: *** 1% significance level; ** 5% significance level; * 10% significance level.

The panel logit regression results show that an individual who suffers from chronic illness in one period has a significantly higher probability of retiring in the subsequent year compared to the same individual free of chronic illness. Some of the respondents in the RLMS have been followed throughout several years of the survey.[8] This allows us to use a panel logit regression in order to assess the impact of chronic illness in one year on the probability of retirement in the subsequent year. In this case we assess the effects of chronic illness on the probability of entering retirement in the next year, not the effect on the probability of retiring in a given year after first employment. Otherwise, the set of explanatory variables to be controlled for is identical to the Cox model. The results (Table 4.3) show a very similar pattern to those based on the Cox regressions (Table 4.2), with only minor differences. In particular, chronic illness emerges as a highly significant predictor of subsequent retirement. Given the different methodology, this result provides a more reliable basis for claiming causality between chronic illness and the probability of retirement. The magnitude of its effect is large compared to other variables in the model.

In either approach, the effect of chronic illness is found to vary with income: the lower the income the more chronic illness affects the retirement decision.

---

[8] This is the "panel" component of the RLMS, which in principle offers important opportunities for testing hypotheses that involve a causal perspective. One shortcoming of this panel dimension is that it does not feature a true panel design, as households that moved from their dwelling and individuals who moved from their household are not followed. In any case, the effect of attrition is relatively modest and is highest for the respondents from the metropolitan areas of Moscow and St Petersburg.

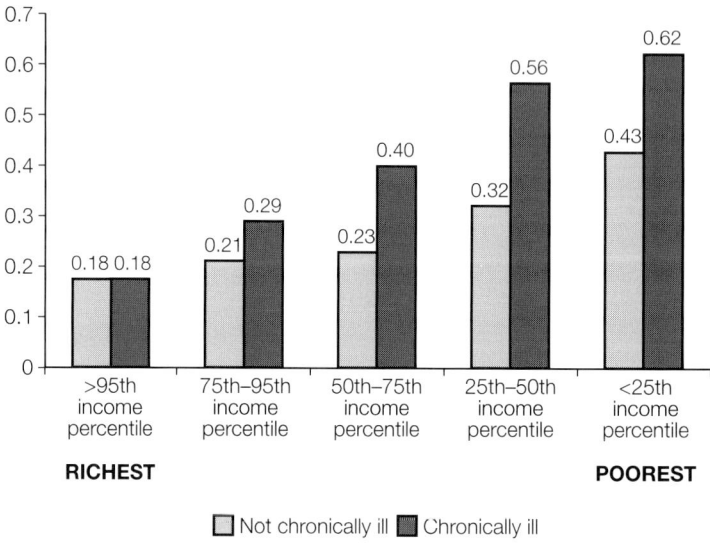

Figure 4.3 *Average predicted probability of retiring in the subsequent period, hypothetical male at varying income levels: based on panel logit model*

Note: Results refer to the hypothetical individual described in the text.
Source: Calculations based on RLMS rounds 9–11.

This implies that less-affluent people carry a double burden of ill-health: first, they are more likely to suffer from chronic illness; second, once they fall ill, they suffer worse economic consequences than rich people – a feature that tends to perpetuate socioeconomic disadvantage.[9] Technically speaking, this result is reflected in the statistically significant interaction term between income and chronic illness in the regression models. As far as Cox regression is concerned, this can be illustrated by comparing the effect of chronic illness in the hypothetical individual described above to another individual with the same characteristics but with an income of 50% of the median: he will retire, on average, at 58.8 years without a chronic illness but at 56.3 if a chronic illness is present – 2.5 years earlier, as opposed to 2 years earlier in the case of the richer individual. This result exemplifies the gradient of the impact on the basis of the panel logit model: among males with a very high income, the presence of a chronic illness has no effect on retirement age, while men just below the average of the income distribution have a 24% higher probability of retiring early compared to their healthy counterparts (Figure 4.3).

---

[9] Note that we are not able to explore a similar variation of the effect of ill-health across the income scale in the wage and earnings regressions presented above. This would require a different approach, for instance a quantile regression (see, for example, Rivera and Currais (1999) for an application of quantile regressions relating to Brazil).

4.1.1.4 The impact of alcohol consumption on the probability of being fired

Heavy alcohol consumption is arguably the most important proximate cause of adult mortality in the Russian Federation. Furthermore, several studies in other developed countries have shown that heavy consumption has a negative impact on earnings, incomes and wages, because it reduces individual productivity and may create problems with working arrangements for the employer.[10] In this subsection we apply this idea to the available Russian data by exploring whether alcohol consumption in one year (2001, round 11 of RLMS) increases the risk of job loss in the subsequent year (2002, round 12). The rationale for this exercise is that job loss would be a natural consequence of an appreciable reduction in individual productivity.

We find that one negative economic impact of severe alcohol consumption is that it significantly increases the probability of losing one's job. Using a panel probit model and controlling for gender, age, education, work experience, wage rate and the ownership type of the employing organization, we find that alcohol has a positive and statistically significant effect on the probability of being fired, even if its size appears relatively small (see Box 4.3). The small size may reflect the simplified structure of the estimated model. Further research would be necessary to disentangle alcohol's complex but no doubt important effects on the Russian labour market.

Box 4.3 *Technical details and results of panel probit model on the probability of being fired*

> We estimated a probit model of the probability of being "fired", which we made
> dependent on gender, age (in months), wage rate, possession of a high-school
> diploma, post-secondary years of schooling, work experience, type of enterprise
> ownership (state, foreigners, private Russian owners) and, finally, daily alcohol
> consumption (in grams of pure alcohol) and squared daily alcohol consumption.
> The dummy variable "fired" was defined such that it takes the value 1 if an individual
> was employed in round 11 (2002), was not employed in round 12 (2003), and yet
> participated in the workforce in round 12. An alternative definition embodying the
> condition of being unemployed in round 12 produced a very similar identification.
> Through the chosen set-up, we assumed that alcohol consumption had a nonlinear
> effect on the probability of being fired. This supposition was confirmed by other
> analyses. We applied the Huber/White/sandwich estimator of variance in place of the
> traditional calculation to obtain robust standard errors. The results are in Table 4.4.
>
> ▶▶

---

[10] See e.g. Mullahy (1991) and Cercone (1994).

Box 4.3 *(cont.)*

Table 4.4 *Panel probit results on alcohol as a determinant of being fired*

Variable	dF/dx	x-bar
Gender (male = 1)	-.00208	1.54
Age (in months)	.00006 **	472
Monthly normal wage in 2002 roubles	-1.53e-06 **	3422
Secondary school diploma (if yes = 1)	-.0043	1.14
Post-secondary years of schooling	-.0011 **	3.28
Number of working years	-.0010 ***	19.03
Publicly owned firm	-.00208	0.68
Foreign-owned firm	.00852	0.05
Privately owned firm	.00508 *	0.43
Alcohol consumption (per week in grams of pure alcohol)	.00030 **	15.6
Alcohol consumption squared	-2.84e-06 **	1818

Notes: *** 1% significance level; ** 5% significance level; * 10% significance level; dF/dx is for discrete change of dummy variable from 0 to 1; z and P > |z| are the test of the underlying coefficient being 0; Number of obs. = 4173; Wald chi2(11) = 60.89; Log likelihood = -311.60966.

4.1.2 Some wider costs of adult mortality: effect on other household members

So far we have focused on the impact of adult ill-health on the individual directly concerned. This captures only part of the overall effect of adult ill-health, as it leaves out the impact on other people, in particular household members. In this subsection we assess the consequences of an individual's death on surviving household members. We specifically explore two potentially related types of "consequences" of a household member's death: depression and alcohol consumption. Both tend to decrease labour productivity and weaken social ties, so they can be interpreted as relevant proxies of economic outcomes.

The death of a household member was found to increase the probability of suffering from depression by 53%. Again, we exploited the panel dimension of the RLMS, i.e. rounds 11 (2002) and 12 (2003), enabling us to assume a more causal interpretation of the results. We included in the sample only those living in households whose composition remained constant between 2002 and 2003 or was altered because one or more members died. This means that we excluded households who lost members for reasons other than death (e.g. migration, new household formation). Using probit analysis and controlling for relevant variables, we explored the effect of a household member who died in 2002 on the probability that any surviving household member would experience depression in the subsequent year (2003). Results are in Table 4.5. As expected, the probability of depression decreases with the age of the deceased. We also controlled for possible differences in per-capita income in order to check whether depression was related to this factor rather than to the death per se. It appears that differences in per-capita income do not affect the probability of depression.

Table 4.5 *Regression results on the effect of a household member's death on depression*

Variable	dF/dx	x-bar
Gender (male = 1)	-.00208	1.54
Age (in months)	.00006 **	472
Wage rate in 2002 roubles	-1.53e-06 **	3422
Secondary-school diploma (yes = 1)	-.0043	1.14
Post-secondary years of schooling	-.0011 **	3.28
Number of working years	-.0010 ***	19.03
Publicly owned firm	-.00208	0.68
Foreign-owned firm	.00852	0.05
Privately owned firm	.00508 *	0.43
Pure alcohol consumption in grams per week	.00030 **	15.6
Alcohol consumption squared	-2.84e-06 **	1818

Notes: *** 1% significance level; ** 5% significance level; * 10% significance level; Number of obs. = 8113;
LR chi2(9) = 321.50; Log likelihood = -3740.8969.

Alcohol consumption was found to increase by about 10 g per day as a consequence of a death in the household. If the deceased was employed, then the survivor's alcohol consumption increased 25 g per day. Using the same two years, we employed a tobit model including essentially the same control variables as in the depression model. Surprisingly, if the deceased was the household head, there was no independent impact, at least not in the short term that we examined. Detailed results are in Table 4.6.

Table 4.6 *Regression results on alcohol consumption in response to a household member's death*

Variable	Coefficient
Gender (male = 1)	36.47 ***
Age (in months)	-0.01 ***
Employed (yes = 1)	23.21 ***
Difference in per-capita income (after and before death)	0.0005 ***
High-school diploma (yes = 1)	10.75 ***
Number of deceased household members throughout the past year	10.55 **
Number of deceased household members who were household heads	4.40
Number of deceased employed household members	25.19 *
Constant	-44.95 ***

Notes: *** 1% significance level; ** 5% significance level; * 10% significance level; Number of obs. = 8170;
3677 left-censored observations at alcohol<=0; 4493 uncensored observations; LR chi2(8) = 1002.07; Log
likelihood = -26843.276.

4.1.3 The effect of chronic illness on income

Chronic illness has had a negative impact on household incomes in the Russian Federation, particularly in the period 1998–2002. In order to deal with some technical constraints on estimating the causal effect of health on economic outcomes – mainly the issue of endogeneity of the health proxy used – we employed a strategy that differs from that used in our other analyses for the present study.[11] We used a difference-in-differences estimator combined with a propensity score-matching technique, applied to the RLMS surveys from 1994 to 2002. Essentially this technique allowed us to compare pairs of households that were identical except for the presence of health problems. Details of the methodology and the results are in Box 4.4.

Using a two-step procedure, we find chronic illness to contribute to an annual loss of 5.6% of per-capita median income for a hypothetical individual with given characteristics.[12] The first step confirmed a negative effect of poor health (in general) on household income. This effect is greater in 1998–2002 than before the Russian financial crisis. We then used a more detailed logit model to assess the extent to which chronic illness increases the likelihood of experiencing adverse health events. These steps show that chronic illness increases the risk of health problems. Combining the effect of chronic illness and poor health on income then gives the overall indirect impact of chronic illness on household income.

Box 4.4 *Technical details and results of household income impact*

To address the endogeneity problems involved in estimating the effect of health on economic outcomes, we used a strategy that does not employ instrumental variables. A difference-in-differences estimator combined with a propensity score-matching technique is described in Rosenbaum and Rubin (1983) and Heckman, Ichimura and Todd (1997). With this approach, every household experiencing a health problem is matched to a similar household not having health problems. Similarity is defined in terms of a propensity score, i.e. the propensity of experiencing an adverse health event given the household characteristics (for instance whether the household members suffer from chronic illness). By comparing the experiences of two similar households in this way, we can identify the causal effect of health on income. The logic is essentially that of comparing two groups that differ only in relation to the variable of interest. This strategy makes it possible to separate the impact of individual health from other contingent effects.

The results (Table 4.7) show the effect on total income of two different events related to poor health: generic health problems and hospitalization. We devised two separate estimates for the periods 1994–1998 and 1998–2002 to capture the differences between the period immediately before the economic crisis, which began in 1998, and the period after the crisis start. The results irrefutably confirm a negative effect of poor health on household economic well-being: the effect is greater in the later period.

➤➤

---

[11] In the previous sections we tried to address endogeneity either by exploring the lagged effect of ill-health on a specific economic outcome using panel regressions or by applying an instrumental variable estimation in the cross-section regressions. (In one case we also used the instrumental variable estimation in the panel context.)

[12] The household characteristics are: in urban areas, with no smokers and no ex-smokers, no people aged over 60 or below 14, with at least two workers and at least one person who has a high-school diploma.

Table 4.7 *Results from difference-in-differences estimator combined with propensity score technique: effect of adverse health on total income for different periods*

	Total income		
	1994–1998	*1998–2002*	*1994–2002*
Health problems	-22.255	-135.98***	-83.147***
Hospitalization	-136.19***	-105.83***	-82.30***

Note: *** 1% significance level.

To estimate the specific impact of chronic diseases we used a logit model to assess whether and to what extent chronic illness increases the likelihood of experiencing adverse health events. The corresponding results are not reported here, but are available from the authors. The results show that chronic illness increases the risk of health problems as well as of hospitalization and of undergoing a surgical procedure.

Our results confirm that chronic illness *does* indirectly and negatively affect the economic well-being of Russian households, especially since the economic crisis in 1998. But what can we say about the magnitude of the effect? It is not possible to provide a comprehensive answer since the risk of health problems depends not only on the presence of chronically ill people in the household, but also on other factors: number of smokers, household size, number of older people, etc. However, we can provide a specific answer for a specific population: households in urban areas, with no smokers or ex-smokers, no one over 60 or below 14, with at least two workers and at least one person who has a high-school diploma. For this restricted population the average difference in the probability of having health problems between households with chronically ill members and those without is 0.219. The difference in the probability of being hospitalized is 0.038, and the difference in the probability of undergoing a surgical operation is 0.018. Multiplying these differences by the effect of health problems, hospitalization and surgical operation on economic outcomes gives the indirect effect of chronic illness on income. The effect corresponds to 5.6% of median per-capita income.

We have so far demonstrated various channels through which health has had an impact on various economic outcomes in the Russian Federation. This is in line with findings from an increasing body of literature on health and the economy in other countries, both wealthier and less affluent. In each estimate presented here, the results proved statistically highly significant, and where size could be assessed, it is notable.

Section 4.2 looks ahead and asks, "what would the economic benefits to the economy be if the adult disease burden due to NCDs and injuries were reduced by a certain extent over a defined period of time?".

4.2 If health were improved, what macroeconomic benefits would result?

Here we estimate the macroeconomic benefits of reducing mortality rates due to NCDs and injuries among Russian adults and find that they would be substantial, irrespective of the evaluation method. The substantial and certain economic benefit would occur despite the fact that we focus only on the effect of mortality reductions, setting aside the additional impact of the potential associated morbidity reduction. Our main findings are detailed below.

- The static economic benefit – valuing a life year lost by one GDP per capita – of gradually bringing the Russian Federation's adult NCD and injury mortality rates down to current EU15 average rates by the year 2025 is estimated to be between 3.6% and 4.8% of the 2002 Russian GDP.

- The broader "welfare" benefits – valuing a life year by a more broadly defined "value of life" estimate – of achieving current EU15 average rates by 2025 are estimated to be as high as 29% of the 2002 Russian GDP.

- The dynamic benefits, i.e. the effect on economic growth rates, are massive and growing over time. Even if the future returns are discounted to the starting-year value (2002), they represent a multiple of the static GDP effects.

This section proposes different ways of looking at the country-wide impact of health on the Russian economy. We distinguish between static (Section 4.2.1) and dynamic cost estimates (Section 4.2.2). The static cost estimates serve an illustrative purpose and are easier to calculate, while the slightly more complex dynamic cost estimates that assess the impact of health on economic growth present a more complete macroeconomic impact assessment and should be of greatest interest to policy-makers. We also look at the static welfare benefits to do justice to the fact that quality of life is more important than the quantity of goods produced.

4.2.1 The benefits of reducing NCD and injury mortality: a simple static calculation

The first step in evaluating the economic benefits of future mortality scenarios is to define the mortality scenarios themselves. To do so, we followed a deliberately simple approach. We defined three different scenarios for the future development of adult mortality (ages 15–64) between 2002 (the most recent year for which the WHO Mortality Database provides data) and 2025. Focusing only on the impact of NCDs and injuries, we included only changes in adult mortality that are driven by the evolution of adult NCD and injury mortality rates.[13] Hence, our starting point is the definition of three NCD and injury mortality scenarios. Once we define the starting conditions for the models, we can assess future trends by inserting estimated changes in adult mortality rates in the different scenarios.

Scenario 1: Optimistic scenario

This scenario assumes that policies are adopted that bring about a decline in Russian mortality rates from NCDs and injuries to the most recent available level for the 15 countries belonging to the EU prior to May 2004. This corresponds to an annual rate of reduction of 4.6% for NCDs and 6.6% for injuries.

Scenario 2: Intermediate scenario

This scenario assumes that policies are adopted that achieve half the improvement seen in the optimistic scenario. It assumes an annual reduction of 2.3% for NCDs and 3.3% for injuries.

Scenario 3: Status quo

In this scenario, the 2002 level of adult mortality rate from NCDs and injuries in the Russian Federation is assumed to remain constant until 2025. One might object that this is unnecessarily pessimistic as NCD and injury mortality are expected to decline simply as an almost automatic response to the very positive recent (and perhaps future) economic development record, even if no specific additional efforts are undertaken to improve adult health. The future trends cannot be known, but Figure 4.4 shows that (a) the long-term increasing trend of noncommunicable (in particular cardiovascular) disease mortality and injury-related mortality over the past decades leaves very limited hope for a sudden or even gradual reversal of these trends, assuming no change in health/economic policy; and (b) these cause-specific mortality rates have increased significantly in recent years, despite particularly strong economic growth. For these reasons, a scenario where the relevant cause-specific mortality rates would remain at their 2002 levels is considered modestly optimistic.

The effect that each of these scenarios would have on adult mortality rates is illustrated in Figure 4.5, assuming other cause-specific adult mortality rates remain constant.

---

[13] In doing so, we are *understating* the broader health impact that eventual broad-based health interventions are likely to have.

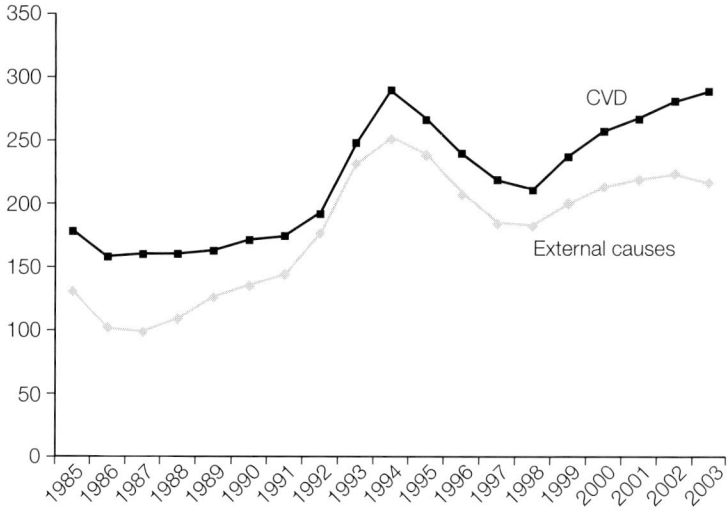

Figure 4.4 *Standardized death rates due to CVD and external causes in the Russian Federation (age 0–64, per 100 000)*

Note: CVD: cardiovascular disease.
Source: WHO Regional Office for Europe European Health for All database 2006.

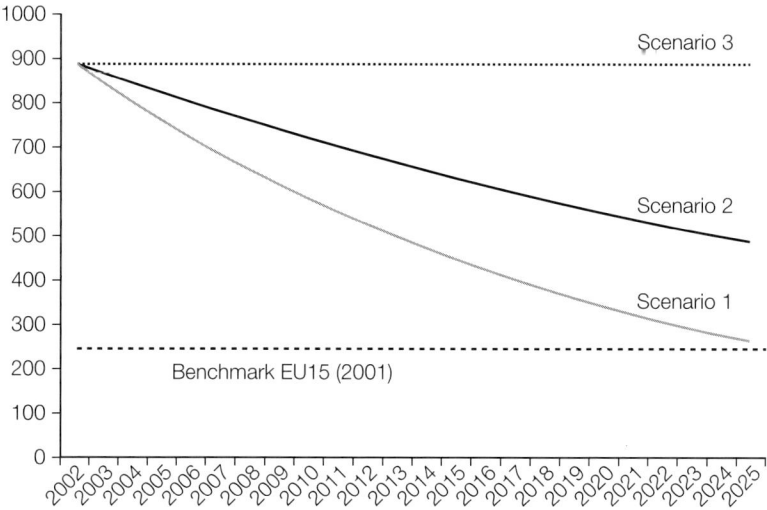

Figure 4.5 *Three scenarios for Russian adult NCD and injury mortality rates (2002–2025) and those of the EU Member States before May 2004 (2001) (age 15–64, per 1000)*

Notes: EU15: Member States belonging to the EU before 1 May 2004; Scenarios are based on the assumptions outlined in the text.
Source: Table 4.8 for initial values and EU15 benchmark.

Table 4.8 *Cause-specific adult death rates in the Russian Federation and EU Member States before May 2004 (age 15–64, per 100 000)*

	Russian Federation	EU15	Death rates as a % of EU15
Noncommunicable diseases	605	206	294%
Injuries	281	58	484%
Cardiovascular diseases	348	37	941%

Notes: Russian rates refer to 2002; EU15 (Member States belonging to the EU before 1 May 2004) rates refer to 2001 or latest available year; The EU15 average is population weighted.
Source: WHO Regional Office for Europe 2006.

None of these scenarios is based on the detailed modelling of the impact of specific policy interventions; this remains a topic for further research. All that matters for our purposes in this study is that the chosen scenarios can be considered to be plausible, i.e. based on the mortality reductions that other western or northern European countries have achieved over the decades. While the most ambitious scenario is indeed very ambitious, it has been achieved in the past (for example the North Karelian and Finnish experiences (World Bank 2005)). Readers will note that the actual levels of the mortality rates foreseen in each of these scenarios are less relevant than the difference between them: the difference between any two scenarios determines the opportunity cost or benefit of the respective scenarios.

Table 4.8 shows the actual mortality rates from NCDs and injury in the Russian Federation (2002) and in the 15 countries belonging to the EU prior to May 2004 (2001). We added CVD mortality for illustrative purposes, as it accounts for the greatest share of total adult NCD mortality. Russian rates are a multiple of the European ones, and the difference is particularly great in the case of CVD mortality.

Next, we undertook a basic economic evaluation to explore the effects of the different scenarios in relation to potential policies to reduce NCDs and injuries up to the year 2025. To evaluate the different scenarios, we use first a "narrow" approach – using foregone production, i.e. GDP per capita – and then a broader perspective to capture the value of living longer without illness.

In what follows we illustrate different ways of assessing the static economic benefits of pursuing the most optimistic and intermediate scenarios compared to the status quo scenario. The first method uses the value of per-capita production (GDP per capita) as the value of a year of adult life lost. This is admittedly a crude (as it lacks a profound theoretical basis), yet not uncommon,[14] way of valuing mortality reductions. The second approach rests on a sound theoretical welfare basis, recognizing that the true cost of a year of life lost greatly exceeds foregone output.

---

[14] The Commission on Macroeconomics and Health also applies a version of this methodology (see CMH 2001, p. 103).

Table 4.9 *Economic benefit estimation for most optimistic scenario*

	Non-communicable diseases	Injuries	Noncommun. diseases + injuries	Cardio-vascular diseases
(A) Zero growth in GDP per capita Present value of benefits 2002–2025 (in million US$ PPP)	286.54	139.75	426.29	176.31
Share of benefits in 2002 GDP (%)	2.42	1.18	3.60	1.49
(B) 3% p.a. growth in GDP per capita Present value of benefits 2002–2025 (in million US$ PPP)	341.26	165.44	506.71	207.53
Share of benefits in 2002 GDP (%)	2.88	1.40	4.27	1.75
(C) 5% p.a. growth in GDP per capita Present value of benefits 2002–2025 (in million US$ PPP)	387.07	186.85	573.91	233.41
Share of benefits in GDP (%)	3.26	1.58	4.84	1.97

Notes: Future benefits are discounted to the present at a 3% rate p.a. (per annum (year)); PPP: purchasing power parity (i.e. real GDP (gross domestic product) per capita).

Static GDP effects

The static economic benefit of gradually bringing the adult NCD and injury mortality rates down to match the current rates for the 15 Member States belonging to the EU prior to 1 May 2004 by the year 2025 (i.e. the optimistic scenario) is estimated to be between 3.6% and 4.8% of the 2002 Russian GDP. Our analysis of the two more optimistic scenarios includes three subscenarios – A, B, and C – each varying with its own assumed future growth path. The higher the future GDP, the more production would be foregone due to a life year lost, and by implication the benefits of reducing mortality would be greater. Under this approach, each year saved (compared to the status quo) was valued by the projected per-capita GDP for the year in which the "saving" occurs. To be able to compare the different future income streams, we calculated the 2002 present value of future values by applying the commonly used discount rate of 3%. Table 4.9 and Table 4.10 report the benefits in both absolute dollars and as a share of GDP for the optimistic scenarios. Again, we include a column that examines the reduction in adult CVD mortality.[15]

It is highly probable that the actual economic gain from reducing future mortality is larger than the static gains calculated above. If dynamic effects exist, they are bound to be larger than any static effect, as even a marginal dynamic impact will outgrow any static gain over time. Substantial empirical evidence shows that health *does* have a positive impact on economic growth and consequently

---

[15] As in the case of NCDs and injuries, we postulate that Russian CVD rates reach the latest rates for the 15 countries belonging to the EU prior to 1 May 2004 by 2025. CVD accounts for the greatest share of the NCD burden.

Table 4.10 *Economic benefit estimation for intermediate scenario*

	Non-communicable diseases	Injuries	Noncommun. diseases + injuries	Cardio-vascular diseases
(A) Zero growth in GDP per capita Present value of benefits 2002–2025				
(in million US$ PPP)	152.17	96.37	248.54	154.74
Share of benefits in 2002 GDP (%)	1.3	0.8	2.1	1.3
(B) 3% p.a. growth in GDP per capita Present value of benefits 2002–2025				
(in million US$ PPP)	229.74	144.90	374.64	231.46
Share of benefits in 2002 GDP (%)	1.9	1.2	3.2	2.0
(C) 5% p.a. growth in GDP per capita Present value of benefits 2002–2025				
(in million US$ PPP)	304.54	191.58	496.12	305.06
Share of benefits in GDP (%)	2.6	1.6	4.2	2.6

Notes: Future benefits are discounted to the present at a 3% rate p.a. (per annum (year)); GDP: gross domestic product; PPP: purchasing power parity.

entails positive dynamic effects on the macroeconomy. The size of the potential dynamic impact of health on the Russian economy is explored in more detail in Section 4.2.2. The Subsection "Static welfare effects" turns to a broader view of the economic assessment while retaining the static perspective. This broader view recognizes that the ultimate goal of economic policy is not the maximization of GDP but of social welfare. (While imperfect, GDP is used simply because it is the most common proxy for social welfare.) In order to assess the broader economic (i.e. welfare) effects of health improvements, it is necessary to translate health improvements into a monetary measure of welfare; the approach described next.

Static welfare effects

Several prominent economists, as well as leading international financial organizations (World Bank, International Monetary Fund (IMF)), have measured the economic cost of mortality using a broader concept than GDP per capita. The new approach starts from the uncontroversial recognition that GDP is an imperfect measure of social welfare, because it fails to incorporate the value of health. The true purpose of economic activity is the maximization of social welfare, not the production of goods alone. Since health is an important component of properly defined social welfare, measuring the economic cost of mortality only in terms of foregone GDP leaves out a potentially major part of its "true economic" impact, i.e. its impact on social welfare.

Even without a market price, health is highly valued – more than most market or other non-market goods. Health is not already incorporated in the measurement of GDP because it is not a market product and consequently has no market price.[16] Yet having no market price does not mean health has no value. When asked, people are ready to pay substantially for better and longer health, so they must attribute some implicit value to health. This value is high, but not infinite, since people are not generally willing to give up everything in exchange for better health.[17]

One way to make the high value attributed to health more explicit is to measure the extent to which one would be willing to trade health for specific market goods for which a price exists. Willingness-to-pay (WTP) studies undertake this measurement. WTP can be inferred from risk premiums in the job market: jobs that entail health risks, such as mining, pay more in the form of a risk premium. A large number of WTP studies now make it possible to calculate the "value of a statistical life" (VSL), which can be used to value changes in mortality. Usher (1973) first introduced the value of mortality reductions into national income accounting. He did so by generating estimates of the growth in "full income", a concept that captures changes in life expectancy by including them in an assessment of economic welfare, for six political entities (Canada, Chile, France, Japan, Sri Lanka, and Taiwan, China) during the middle decades of the 20th century. For the higher-income entities, about 30% of the growth of full income resulted from declines in mortality. Estimates of changes in full income are typically generated by adding the value of changes in annual mortality rates (calculated using VSL figures) to changes in annual GDP per capita. Even these full-income estimates are conservative, including only the value of changes in mortality while excluding the total value of improvements to health.

For the United States, Nordhaus (2003) rediscovered Usher's pioneering work and found that the economic value of increases in longevity since the early 1900s roughly equals the value of measured growth in non-health goods and services. Nordhaus tested the hypothesis that improvements in health status made a major contribution to economic wealth (defined as full income) over the 20th century. A more detailed assessment reveals that "health income" probably contributed to changes in full income somewhat more than non-health goods and services before 1950 and marginally less than non-health goods and services afterwards. If the results of this and other related papers (e.g. Cutler and Richardson 1997; Miller 2000; Costa and Kahn 2004; Crafts 2003;

---

[16] The health care inputs included in the measurement of GDP represent only a small share of the true value of health, as argued here.

[17] We are referring to situations where people face marginal trade-offs between health and other goods, not the far less representative situation where people face immediate death, the prospect of which would increase the readiness to pay.

Viscusi and Aldy 2003) are confirmed, then the role of health should be reconsidered: the social productivity of spending on health (via the health system and other sectors that impact on health) may be many times greater than that of other forms of investment.

Applying this approach to the evaluation of the "welfare" benefits from achieving the most optimistic scenario results in a calculated benefit as high as 29% of the 2001/2002 GDP for the 15 Member States belonging to the EU prior to 1 May 2004. It is straightforward to apply the approach to assess the welfare benefits of reducing adult mortality in the Russian Federation. The critical input is a value of a statistical life for the Russian Federation. The principle in developing such estimates is to ensure that the lower boundary of plausible estimates cannot be challenged. Real values will certainly be higher; however, the key issue is the minimal plausible figure. For the purpose of the present calculations, we used a very conservative estimate of US$ 500 000 for the value of a statistical life in the Russian Federation as of 2002. To assess how conservative this is, see Miller (2000). Miller assembled a collection of VSL studies and estimated an equation that would predict the VSL in terms of gross national product (GNP) per capita and some other factors. Applying the parameters to the Russian Federation, he obtained a range of US$ 300 000 to US$ 800 000 with the best estimate being US$ 370 000. However, these figures were based on 1997 GDP data and expressed in 1995 dollars. Between 1997 and 2003/2004, Russian GDP increased by 30%. An updated VSL would be US$ 500 000 in 1995 dollars. Inflation in the United States between 1995 and 2004 has an accumulated value of 18%, so in 2004 dollars, VSL in the Russian Federation would be US$ 590 000. Thus, the US$ 500 000 used here is certainly a lower bound. Based on a review of existing VSL studies, Crafts (2003) assumed that a conventional estimate of a country's VSL equals 132 times the GDP per capita. For the Russian Federation this would give a 2002 VSL of 132 times US$ 8230, totalling US$ 1 086 360, which is approximately double the estimate in this report. This calculation does, however, assume a unitary income elasticity of VSL; a result that other authors reject in favour of an income elasticity below 1 (see, for example, Viscusi and Aldy 2003), which would tend to reduce the VSL of countries with a lower GDP per capita. Yet even in this case, our estimates remain the lower bound of the range of possible estimates.

Table 4.11 summarizes the results from the welfare benefits estimation of scenarios 1 and 2, assuming a Russian VSL of US$ 500 000. In our calculations we used the same discount rate (3%) for future benefits as were used in the calculations that generated the figures in Table 4.9 and Table 4.10. We assume that the VSL remains constant over the period 2002–2025, which is in line

Table 4.11 *Welfare benefits of most optimistic and intermediate scenarios*

	Non-communicable diseases	Injuries	Noncommun. diseases + injuries	Cardio-vascular diseases
Most optimistic scenario				
Present value of benefits per capita (in US$ PPP)	1512	866	2377	1242
Share of benefits in 2002 GDP (%)	18.4	10.5	28.9	15.1
Intermediate scenario				
Present value of benefits per capita (in US$ PPP)	919	565	1484	876
Share of benefits in 2002 GDP (%)	11.2	6.9	18.0	10.6

Notes: GDP: gross domestic product; PPP: purchasing power parity.

with the literature if GDP per capita also remains constant (sub-scenario A in Table 4.9). If GDP per capita grows over time, the VSL will increase in future years, too, thereby even further increasing the welfare benefits to health.

One interpretation of the figures in Table 4.11 is that in 2002 the average Russian would have been willing to pay US$ 1512 if by so doing he could have expected to experience a reduction in the risk of noncommunicable mortality of the scale set out in the most optimistic scenario. Not surprisingly, the estimated welfare benefits are a multiple of the narrower returns in the previous GDP-based calculations. Specifically, the accumulated effects of reductions in mortality from NCD and injuries are approximately 10 times higher than when using the narrow concept.

Subsection 4.2.2 assesses the likely impact of the three adult mortality scenarios on economic growth, complementing the static GDP analysis presented in this subsection.

4.2.2 Dynamic effects: the impact of adult health on economic growth

Recent worldwide empirical evidence strongly suggests that health is a robust determinant of economic growth. Such growth is driven by effects on savings (Bloom, Canning and Graham 2003), on human capital investment (Kalemi-Ozcan, Ryder and Weil 2000), on labour market participation (Thomas 2001), on foreign direct investment (Alsan, Bloom and Canning 2004), and on productivity growth (Bloom, Canning and Sevilla 2002). The combined effects of health on economic growth are confirmed in theoretic and empirical work by Barro (1996); Bhargava, Jamison and Murray (2001); Bloom, Canning and Sevilla (2001); Jamison, Lau and Wang (2004), and many more. Studies examining the impact of health on income levels or income growth differ substantially in terms of country samples, time frames, control variables, functional forms, data definitions and configurations, and estimation techniques. Nevertheless, parameter estimates of the effects of life expectancy on economic growth have been remarkably comparable and robust across studies, notwithstanding the observation that the empirical growth regression results are generally not very robust, given the high degree of multicollinearity between many of the explanatory variables used (Levine and Renelt 1992; Sala-I-Martin, Doppelhofer and Miller 2004). In some studies, initial health status, typically proxied by life expectancy or adult mortality, proved to be a more significant and more important predictor of subsequent growth than the education indicators employed (Barro 1997). Bhargava, Jamison and Murray (2001), for instance, show in the context of a panel regression that the 5-year growth rate of GDP per capita depends on a country's adult mortality rate, among other factors. They also show that the direction of causality runs *unambiguously* from adult mortality to growth. This subsection applies this empirical relationship to the Russian Federation and then employs the empirical results to project different future pathways in GDP per capita, using the same three scenarios. In doing so, an assumption is made that the empirical regularities that hold in a representative world sample of countries also hold for the Russian Federation (see Box 4.5 for details).

Applied to the specific Russian context, the dynamic benefits of improving adult health, i.e. the effect on economic growth rates, are massive and growing over time. One conservative estimate indicates that while in 2005 the difference in per-capita GDP between the status quo scenario and the most optimistic scenario is only US$ 105–324 (depending on the estimation methodology used), by 2025 this difference would have grown to US$ 2856–9243. Even if these future returns are discounted to the starting-year value, they represent a multiple of the static GDP effects. Figure 4.6 illustrates the predicted path of GDP per capita under the three scenarios, using the very conservative lower bound of the growth estimates calculated. The area between the lines for scenarios 1 and 3 indicates the economic (opportunity) benefit of the optimistic scenario.

Box 4.5 explains the methodology and presents further results.

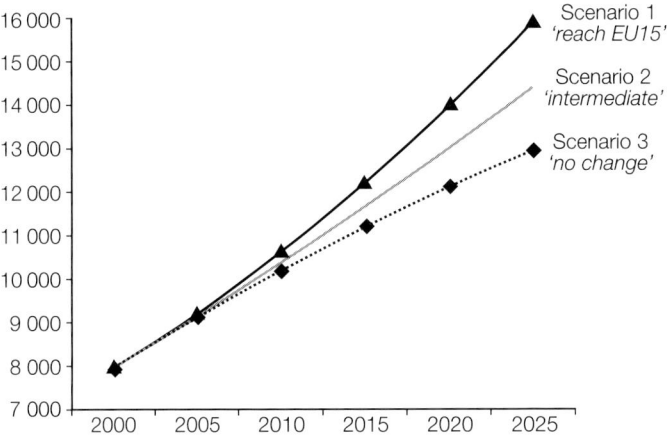

Figure 4.6 *GDP per capita (in US$ PPP) forecasts in the three scenarios*
Notes: GDP: gross domestic product; PPP: purchasing power parity.

Box 4.5 *Technical details and results of economic growth impact estimates*

We start by running a standard pooled OLS panel growth regression for the period 1960–2000. The dependent variable is the annual average of the 5-year growth rate of real GDP per capita. The other explanatory variables are the 5-year time lag of GDP per capita, the lagged fertility rate, the lagged working-age mortality rate,[18] and the Warner-Sachs index of openness.[19] The fertility rate is from the World Development Indicators (World Bank 2004) and the adult mortality rate is constructed from the WHO Mortality Database.

Since OLS panel growth regressions yield downward-biased estimates on the projected growth rate (Trognon 1978), we also apply a fixed effects (FE) estimator on the same regression equation. The FE regression is known to yield upward-biased estimates on the projected growth rate (Nickel 1981). Thus, the unbiased growth path is bounded by the OLS and FE estimates. The regression results of the OLS and FE regressions are shown in Table 4.12.

The growth projections from OLS estimates show that there is a growth rate of 14% on average over a 5-year period, or approximately 3% per annum. Accordingly, the growth projections based on FE estimates suggest even an annual growth rate of approximately 7%. The results, shown in Table 4.12, show a convergence rate of 14% using OLS or even 35% with an FE estimator, well above the 2% that is well

▶▶

---

[18] Working age is assumed to be between 15 and 64.
[19] This variable is a time-invariant dummy variable with value 1 if an economy has been considered as open during 1965 and 1990. See Sachs and Warner (1995).

Table 4.12 *Growth regression results*

Dependent variable: GDP per capita	OLS	FE
Lagged GDP per capita	.86*** (.02)	.65*** (.05)
Lagged fertility rate	-.05 (.03)	-.17*** (.06)
Openness	.16***	(.02) -
Lagged adult mortality rate	-.08** (.04)	-.18*** (.06)
R²	0.97	0.98
No. of observations	302	332

Notes: Heteroscedasticity-consistent standard errors in parentheses; *, **, *** denote significance at the 10%, 5%, and 1% levels, respectively; constant terms are not reported.

Sources: GDP (gross domestic product) data are from Penn World Data 6.0 (available at http://pwt.econ.upenn.edu/); Openness is a time-invariant dummy variable between 1965 and 1990 from Gallup and Sachs (1999), available at http://www.cid.harvard.edu/ ciddata/ciddata.html; the fertility rate is from World Bank (2004).

known in the empirical growth literature. However, as Islam (1995) noted, convergence rates increase dramatically in a panel data context. The long-run convergence rate is then mixed with business cycle effects. Concerning the variable of interest in this study, the lagged adult mortality rate is found to be highly significant for both estimators with a negative sign as expected. Hence, the larger the mortality rate, the lower the GDP per-capita growth.

Next, these alternative growth regressions are used to predict Russian GDP per capita up to the year 2025. This requires an assumption about the future path of the fertility rate, which was taken from United Nations Population Division forecasts. The openness status of the Russian economy is assumed to stay constant over the next 20 years as the key question for this study relates to different mortality scenarios. An increase in openness would not change results dramatically, although the growth path would become somewhat steeper.

As for the adult mortality scenarios, we use the same ones here as those described above (Figure 4.5). Based on these scenarios, a forward prediction is carried out separately on the OLS and FE estimates. The results are shown in Figure 4.7.

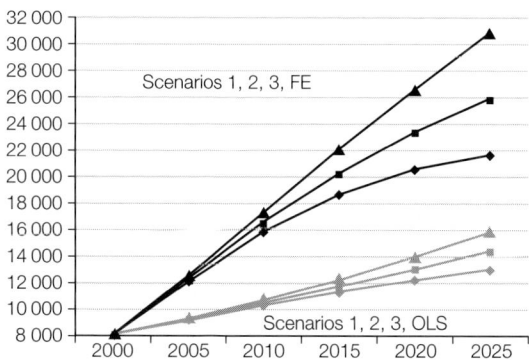

Figure 4.7 *GDP per capita (in US$ PPP) forecasts based on OLS and FE regression*

Notes: OLS: ordinary least squares; FE: fixed effect; PPP: purchasing power parity.
Source: Authors' calculations based on model presented in Table 4.12.

Box 4.5 *(cont.)*

As Figure 4.7 illustrates, the predicted per-capita GDP path is highly dependent on the choice of estimation methodology. As expected, the FE estimates produce a steeper growth path than the OLS estimates, and the "true" effect will lie somewhere in between. In either type of estimate, however, there is a sizeable impact of the reduction of mortality rates on future incomes, and the effect grows over time. While in 2005 the difference in the per-capita GDP between the first (*"Do nothing"*) and the third (*"Committed action"*) is only US$ 115 in the OLS estimation (and US$ 354 in the FE estimates), by 2025 this difference would have grown to US$ 3151 (respectively US$ 10 280). Even if these future returns are discounted to the starting-year value, they make the static GDP effects calculated in the narrower approach of the previous section appear tiny.

Chapter 5
Further action

Although it achieved much in the first half of the 20th century, ensuring that basic health care was delivered to a poor and widely dispersed population, the Soviet health care system failed to adapt to changing circumstances. From the mid-1960s onwards, diversion of resources to the military–industrial complex, coupled with the stifling effect of communist ideology on innovation, meant that the USSR was unable to take advantage of the developments in pharmaceuticals, technology, and evidence-based medicine that were of growing importance in the West. This was apparent from an analysis of avoidable mortality rates. These are deaths from causes (for example diabetes or asthma) that should not occur prematurely in the presence of timely and effective care. Death rates from these causes in the USSR were comparable to those in western countries in the mid-1960s but subsequently, as they fell rapidly in the West, they remained stubbornly high in the USSR (Andreev et al. 2003).

In the post-independence period, the Russian Federation, like its former-Soviet neighbours, has undergone a series of health care reforms (Tragakes and Lessof 2003). It has made a relatively successful transition to a funding model based on health insurance, although a significant minority of already marginalized people remain outside the system (Balabanova, Falkingham and McKee 2003). It is, however, the delivery of care that has proven much more resilient to change. The design, configuration, and geographical distribution of many health facilities reflects the Soviet period, in which large numbers of staff substituted, to some degree, for the lack of modern technology, in both clinical and support services. Soviet medicine was largely isolated from developments elsewhere and even now many clinical practices are incompatible with scientific evidence. Although strenuous efforts have been made to retrain the health workforce, the experience with family medicine, where efforts have been concentrated, indicates the scale of the challenge ahead (Rese et al. 2005).

Yet while there is still much to be done to ensure that the health care system is able to address the needs of the Russian population, in particular to prevent the consequences of existing disease, such as better control of high blood pressure, the greatest gains are likely to be upstream, deriving from the design and implementation of healthy public policies. The Government of the Russian Federation is currently developing a federal programme for the prevention and control of the NCDs that are the major causes of the poor health of its population. This programme will require the development of policies and strategies at federal level that can complement and enable implementation of priority intervention programmes in regions and municipalities.

There are several areas in which action is urgently needed. The immediate causes of the high level of premature mortality in the Russian Federation, compared with western countries, are CVD and injuries and violence. The major risk factors underlying this high burden of disease in the Russian Federation include hazardous alcohol consumption, smoking, and inadequate diet. Looking ahead, the threat of a marked increase in HIV/AIDS cannot be ignored.

While the health consequences of heavy drinking in the Russian Federation have long been recognized, more recent work is quantifying the scale of this problem. This suggests that at least 40% of deaths in young and middle-aged men can be attributed to hazardous drinking. A particular concern is the widespread consumption of alcohol-containing substances, such as aftershaves and technical spirits that are not intended to be drunk. As they are untaxed, but contain up to 96% ethanol, they are a cheap and easily available source of alcohol for many people (McKee et al. 2005).

Smoking has been common among Russian men for several decades, but less common among Russian women. This is now changing in the face of massive marketing efforts by international tobacco companies, with recent increases among women in rural areas (Bobak et al. 2006). Urgent action is needed if the forthcoming epidemic of smoking-related diseases among Russian women is to be slowed down.

The traditional Russian diet is energy dense, with a high fat content and few vegetables. This is changing as retail distribution systems respond to the incentives created by the market. Thus, it is now possible to get year-round fresh fruit in many places where this was previously impossible. However, the market has also brought threats, in the form of western fast-food outlets. It will be necessary to develop effective, multifaceted nutrition policies that reflect this changing environment.

Finally, there is a need for an appropriate response to the high burden of injury. This is complicated by the diverse forms of violent death, which range from traffic and industrial injuries to homicide. However, as the experience of other countries has shown, with appropriate multi-agency working, much can be done.

As the previous chapters of this report have shown, the economic cost of the high burden of disease in the Russian Federation is great. It will continue to act as a drag on economic growth in the future unless effective action is taken. This chapter can only act as a pointer to what is needed, but it does provide a starting point.

Chapter 6
Conclusions

Policy-makers in the health arena and beyond must certainly garner their resources to meet the growing need for and cost of health care. This report cites previous research showing that NCDs and injuries pose a great threat to Russians. Worse yet, that research shows that NCDs and injuries are killing Russians during their productive years, ages 15–64, and that the prevalence rate is rising markedly. Furthermore, the morbidity and mortality from these causes is significantly greater in the Russian Federation than in other countries.

The high mortality rate, striking people during their working years, is a blow to production, which in turn strikes doubly on economic resources. First, those people who die are not buying and producing goods and services; activities that would contribute to both the economy and Government revenues. Second, surviving family members of people killed by NCDs and injuries draw on Government resources with their needs – as do those household survivors who react to a death in the household by experiencing depression and increased alcohol consumption; risk factors believed to bring on yet more illness and death. Recent medical advancements have supported the health care model where health care systems focus on curing those who fall ill; however, it may be that this model is pursued at the Russian Federation's peril. NCDs and injuries are preventable, and prevention would avoid both the costs of care and the previously noted blows to the economy.

The follow-up question is obvious: how much of these costs could be avoided, either by better prevention or treatment? This report contributes to the previous research in order to provide, with as much accuracy and certainty as possible, likely estimates of the savings that would accrue from improving health. We assessed three plausible scenarios that assume varying levels of success from intervention efforts, to present the range of savings that could be recouped. In this report, we describe as carefully as possible our statistical methods, conservative assumptions and the results from our methods and find little doubt that successful intervention would not only improve the lives of Russians but would also be good for the Russian economy – significantly so.

Our research shows that reducing the Russian Federation's mortality rates from NCDs and injuries to match the EU average rate (for the 15 EU Member States before 1 May 2004) by 2025 (or, more modestly, to half that rate) could contribute markedly to prevent a substantial levelling off of the pace of economic growth in the Russian Federation. Those estimates – which set aside the fact that if mortality rates improve, morbidity rates would likely follow suit and similarly accrue economic benefits – recommend serious consideration by policy-makers to increase health investments in the Russian Federation.

While little is certain in these times of rapidly changing health threats and medical advancements, the policy implication is that investing in adult health is a sound strategy that is likely to yield tangible economic returns (in addition to the welfare benefits) and, given the magnitude of economic benefits that can be expected from improving adult health in the Russian Federation, would produce a significant economic return. The intent of this research is to provide a foundation upon which policy-makers can allocate resources towards the greatest return on investment. We conclude that our research shows that reducing NCDs and injuries may be a very sensible course of action.

Appendix

Description of micro datasets used

Russian Longitudinal Monitoring Survey (RLMS)

The RLMS was conducted with the support and assistance of the World Bank, the United States Agency for International Development (USAID), the National Science Foundation, the National Institute of Health, and the North Carolina Population Center.

The RLMS covers the period from 1992 to 2003, but the survey changed considerably throughout this period: in the first phase (from 1992 to 1994), the main RLMS accomplishment was the creation of the first national sample frame allowing surveys to be representative at national level. More recently, this sample frame has been extended to develop samples representative at the regional and oblast levels (RLMS 1998). For the second phase, covering the period 1994–2003, the emphasis changed from institution-building to providing timely, high-quality information. The survey's main unit of observation is the household. The RLMS covers primarily the European part of the Russian Federation, but the distribution of household size in the sample within urban and rural areas corresponds well to the figures from the 1989 census (for a detailed comparison of the 1989 census and the RLMS, see RLMS (1998)). At each round, data are collected on the household, each household member, and the residential community.

Houscholds were selected on the basis of a multi-stage process, with the households being clustered into primary sampling units ("sites"). Although the target sample size was 4000 households, the number of households drawn into the second phase sample was 4728, in order to allow for a 15% non-response rate. The household response rate in the beginning of the second phase of the RLMS exceeded 80%, and individual questionnaires were obtained from about 97% of the individuals listed in the household rosters.

This dataset lacks a true panel design, as households are not followed if they move from their dwelling, and likewise, individuals who leave a household are not followed. The effect of attrition is relatively modest and has been highest for the respondents from Moscow and St Petersburg.

The information is rich on income and expenditures of households, labour force participation, health conditions, and individual risk factors.

National Survey of Household Welfare and Program Participation

While the RLMS has the advantage of being repeated annually, which allows some comparison over time, the National Survey of Household Welfare and Program Participation (NOBUS) survey, so far only held once, in 2003, covers a far more comprehensive portion of the population. With a sample of about 44 500 households, it is representative both nationally and for 46 larger subjects of the Russian Federation. It captures differing aspects of household welfare and focuses on household access to social services. Its health measurement component, however, is small compared to the RLMS, so a direct comparison to the RLMS results is not possible.

Details of calculations on the costs of absenteeism

Table A.1 Calculation for costs of absenteeism

Year	Gender	Annual average working days missed due to illness	Average annual wage (among all job holders)	Average annual wage (among those absent at least once)	GDP per capita (in current local currency units, in constant 2000 prices)	Average wage loss for a person who was absent the average number of days	Average production loss for a person who was absent the average number of days	Active population	Total income loss (billions)	Total production (GDP) loss (billions)
2000	Male	10.8	26 268	24 576		777	1 480	36 639 000	28.48	54.24
	Female	9.24	15 648	15 864		396	1 266	33 822 000	13.40	42.83
	Total	10.08	20 724	19 992	50 028	572	1 382	70 461 000	40.33	97.35
2001	Male	9.48	32 501	33 994		844	1 373	36 788 000	31.05	50.52
	Female	10.92	20 335	20 046		608	1 582	34 402 000	20.93	54.42
	Total	10.2	26 145	26 062	52 876	731	1 478	71 190 000	52.01	105.19
2002	Male	8.64	37 448	37 929		886	1 318	36 937 000	32.74	48.70
	Female	10.32	23 891	25 146		675	1 575	34 982 000	23.63	55.09
	Total	9.48	30 309	30 763	55 699	787	1 447	71 919 000	56.62	104.04
2003	Male	9.6	40 514	36 851		1066	1 583	37 087 000	39.52	58.72
	Female	9.36	25 552	25 544		655	1 544	35 125 000	23.02	54.22
	Total	9.48	32 503	30 570	60 195	844	1 563	72 212 000	60.96	112.90
Sources:		RLMS	RLMS	RLMS	IMF					

Notes: We used the population average wage in the cost calculations since there were no systematic patterns when comparing population average wage and absentees' average wage; RLMS: Russian Longitudinal Monitoring Survey; IMF: International Monetary Fund; GDP: gross domestic product.

Detailed results on the impact of health on labour supply and productivity

Ordinary least squares (OLS) regressions

Tables A.2 and A.3 report estimates of four models, whose difference is the date of medical diagnosis of diabetes, heart attack, stroke, TB and hepatitis, which are the unique diseases for which the diagnosis date is available in our dataset. It reveals that lung, kidney and spinal disease reduce wage rate, as expected. Surprisingly, chronic lung disease increases labour supply. Recently diagnosed heart attack and TB reduce the wage rate, as expected. Hepatitis diagnosed very early reduces labour supply, while recently diagnosed TB increases labour supply. Indeed, respiratory and lung diseases (such as asthma and bronchitis) seem to have a positive effect on labour supply. A possible rationale for this paradox, which requires more research, is that individuals may seek to augment their revenue to compensate for the additional costs of medical care expenditures they incur.

Instrumental variables regression

The sample used is again that resulting from pooling rounds 9–12 of the RLMS.

Variables in the third column of box A are used as instruments for self-evaluated health status and missed days due to ill-health, respectively (the chosen date of diagnosis for the last five is between 10 and 5 years previously). Table A.5 and Table A.6 report estimates for both the logarithms of wage rate and labour supply, distinguishing by gender. Both indicators negatively affect wage rate and, on the contrary, they have no significant influence on labour supply. A reported good health status increases wage rate by 22% for women and by 18% for men. Similarly, a day missed reduces wage rate by 3.7% in the male subsample and by 5.5% among females.

The Sargan test of overidentification does not reject the hypothesis of exogeneity of the selected instruments. Although this result must be interpreted only as an indication of exogeneity, as the Sargan test has only little power, it supports the Bartel and Taubman (1979) assumption of exogeneity of the health conditions they used in their analysis.

Table A.2 *Independent variables used in the regression analysis (RLMS data)*

Variable	Description	Instrumental variables*
Gender	Gender (male = 1)	
Age	Age	
age2	Age squared	
Highsc	High-school diploma	
Tecdp	Technical or medical diploma	
Insdp	Institute or university diploma	
Gradp	Doctoral degree	
Married	Married	
Tenure	Experience at current workplace	
tenure2	Experience at current workplace squared	
Pjemps	Number of employees in enterprise	
Ncat	Number of children under 7 years	
Private	Private sector	
region_2	Northern and North-western	
region_3	Central and Central Black-Earth	
region_4	Volga-Vaytski and Volga Basin	
region_5	North Caucasian	
region_6	Ural	
region_7	Western Siberian	
region_8	Eastern Siberian and Far Eastern	
Urban	Urban area	
Occupation_2	Professionals (ISCO-88 code)	
Occupation_3	Technicians and associate professionals (ISCO-88 code)	
Occupation_4	Clerks (ISCO-88 code)	
Occupation_5	Service workers and market workers (ISCO-88 code)	
Occupation_6	Skilled agricultural (ISCO-88 code)	
Occupation_7	Craft and related trades (ISCO-88 code)	
Occupation_8	Plant and machine operators and assemblers (ISCO-88 code)	
Occupation_9	Elementary (unskilled) occupations (ISCO-88 code)	
round_10	Year 2001	
round_11	Year 2002	
round_12	Year 2003	
Cheart	Chronic heart disease	X
Clungs	Chronic lung disease	X
Cliver	Chronic liver disease	X
Ckidny	Chronic kidney disease	X
Cgi	Chronic stomach disease	X
Spine	Chronic spine disease	X
Cother	Other chronic diseases	X
diabetes_10	Diabetes diagnosed between 10 and 5 years ago	X
diabetes_20	Diabetes diagnosed between 20 and 10 years ago	
diabetes_5	Diabetes diagnosed less than 5 years ago	
diabetes_b20	Diabetes diagnosed more than 20 years ago	
heart_10	Heart attack diagnosed between 10 and 5 years ago	X
heart_20	Heart attack diagnosed between 20 and 10 years ago	
heart_5	Heart attack diagnosed less than 5 years ago	
heart_b20	Heart attack diagnosed more than 20 years ago	
hepatitis_10	Hepatitis diagnosed between 10 and 5 years ago	X
hepatitis_20	Hepatitis diagnosed between 20 and 10 years ago	
hepatitis_5	Hepatitis diagnosed less than 5 years ago	
hepatitis_b20	Hepatitis diagnosed more than 20 years ago	
stroke_10	Stroke diagnosed between 10 and 5 years ago	X
stroke_20	Stroke diagnosed between 20 and 10 years ago	
stroke_5	Stroke diagnosed less than 5 years ago	
stroke_b20	Stroke diagnosed more than 20 years ago	
tbc_10	Tuberculosis diagnosed between 10 and 5 years ago	X
tbc_20	Tuberculosis diagnosed between 20 and 10 years ago	
tbc_5	Tuberculosis diagnosed less than 5 years ago	
tbc_b20	Tuberculosis diagnosed more than 20 years ago	
healthGOOD	Self-reported good health status	
misseddays	Missed work days due to ill-health	
school_1	High-school diploma completed before 2000	
school_2	Technical or medical diploma completed before 2000	
school_3	Institute or university diploma completed before 2000	
school_4	Doctoral degree completed before 2000	

Note: * With the RLMS data instrumental variables have only been used in the regressions summarized in Table A.5 and Table A.6.

Table A.3 *OLS – dependent variable: log hourly wage rate (2000 prices)*

Variable	The disease was diagnosed... 20 years earlier	10–20 years earlier	5–10 years earlier	0–5 years earlier
gender	.30254066***	.30310181***	.3024037***	.30367693***
age	.03272136***	.03260822***	.03273228***	.03251867***
age2	-.00041325***	-.00041165***	-.00041368***	-.0004103***
highsc	.07731209***	.07729698***	.0775283***	.07760015***
tecdp	.08662943***	.08694422***	.08624272***	.08602663***
insdp	.32191213***	.32172709***	.32240742***	.32086648***
gradp	-.07311596	-.07601234	-.07762188	-.07221849
married	.04515979***	.04471361***	.04424292***	.04513566***
tenure	-.00126128	-.00124136	-.00126923	-.00110397
tenure2	.00011182*	.00011086*	.00011178*	.0001044*
pjemps	9.158e-06***	9.184e-06***	9.16e-06***	9.201e-06***
ncat	-.04025733***	-.04012284***	-.03946076***	-.04009372***
private	.17656016***	.17648686***	.17705347ᴬᴬᴬ	.17630873***
region_2	-.02601835	-.02536182	-.0264554	-.0255168
region_3	-.46472316***	-.46428774***	-.46488513***	-.46488793***
region_4	-.71409733***	-.71366399***	-.7137759***	-.71324021***
region_5	-.61041382***	-.60970428***	-.61063961***	-.60931095***
region_6	-.48056355***	-.48006629***	-.48088991***	-.48145873***
region_7	-.48499262***	-.48461688***	-.48570588***	-.48480409***
region_8	-.29421497***	-.29363089***	-.29479044***	-.29217805***
urban	.43861682***	.43867082***	.4389986***	.44019666***
occupation_2	-.01549473	-.0169319	-.01764095	-.01722858
occupation_3	-.1018942***	-.10313616***	-.10426042***	-.102774***
occupation_4	-.16137001***	-.16203158***	-.16283756***	-.16217807***
occupation_5	-.41726362***	-.41845074***	-.41930993***	-.41848629***
occupation_6	-.46935269***	-.47401677***	-.47384018***	-.47511778***
occupation_7	-.04230204	-.04379586	-.04411402	-.04298466
occupation_8	-.11553389***	-.11695315***	-.11749264***	-.11677098***
occupation_9	-.48967173***	-.48989482***	-.49126905***	-.49107733***
round_10	.17638925***	.17525387***	.17556241***	.17504897***
round_11	.38113833***	.38000061***	.38030253***	.37951903***
round_12	.47109966***	.46966934***	.47030324***	.46988307***
cheart	-.02067898	-.01857795	-.01968821	-.01338115
clungs	-.08023211**	-.07860568**	-.07878113**	-.07764093**
cliver	-.00480458	-.00782106	-.00376398	-.01182401
ckidny	-.04546527*	-.04487214*	-.04552355*	-.0444479*
cgi	.01611436	.01571097	.01533843	.01483718
cspine	-.03773294**	-.03885295**	-.0386692**	-.03875688**
cother	-.02434006	-.02327219	-.02333522	-.02540852
diabetes_b~0	.08708819			
heart_b20	–			
stroke_b20	-.12886329			
tbc_b20	-.11782447			
hepatitis_b20	-.02362581			
diabetes_20		-.08324869		
heart_20		-.06870232		
stroke_20		-.23865608		
tbc_20		-.04481312		
hepatitis_20		.00727449		
diabetes_10			-.03340999	
heart_10			.0153402	
stroke_10			-.2775952	
tbc_10			-.12228027	
hepatitis_10			-.04278534	
diabetes_5				.05831311
Heart_5				-.13975016*
Stroke_5				-.10652745
tbc_5				-.23336728**
hepatitis_5				.10332314
Constant	1.2241776***	1.2269543***	1.226739***	1.2266473***
R2	.3803084	.38032227	.38038093	.3806654
N	11 297	11 297	11 297	11 297

Notes: * p<.1; ** p<.05; *** p<.01.

Table A.4 *OLS – dependent variable: log weekly hours*

Variable	The disease was diagnosed...			
	20 years earlier	10–20 years earlier	5–10 years earlier	0–5 years earlier
gender	.1082822***	.10816178***	.10869426***	.10820324***
age	.01699662***	.01691379***	.01676215***	.01688689***
age2	-.00020535***	-.00020482***	-.00020268***	-.00020421***
highsc	-.01192034	-.01158593	-.01202024	-.01188906
tecdp	.00299955	.0030822	.00286354	.00316107
insdp	.00574539	.00556812	.00571997	.00574958
gradp	.01750542	.01471094	.01609397	.01712725
married	-.02446514***	-.02487114***	-.02475416***	-.02468505***
tenure	-.00206881**	-.00206111**	-.00207175**	-.00207253**
tenure2	.00005766**	.00005736**	.0000583**	.00005743**
pjemps	-8.690e-07***	-8.490e-07***	-8.641e-07***	-8.489e-07***
ncat	.00040164	.00039929	.00030107	.00046486
private	.07633224***	.07656981***	.07671271***	.07617914***
region_2	.06115134***	.06051219***	.0609761***	.06085042***
region_3	.02044861*	.02015783*	.02036473*	.02046827*
region_4	.03674088***	.03693256***	.03682934***	.03713913***
region_5	.07975371***	.07938687***	.07960869***	.08008555***
region_6	.01340273	.01321734	.01336299	.01393258
region_7	.04322431***	.04314116***	.04295671***	.04327367***
region_8	.05036055***	.05051396***	.05041537***	.05130143***
urban	.02271182***	.02296056***	.02270854***	.02260605***
occupation_2	-.17578267***	-.17522752***	-.17577442***	-.1761433***
occupation_3	-.07078628***	-.07051406***	-.07101583***	-.07137268***
occupation_4	-.0686374***	-.0680209***	-.06813237***	-.06915404***
occupation_5	.08926562***	.0897478***	.08947398***	.08936801***
occupation_6	-.02700664	-.02734797	-.02807609	-.02808858
occupation_7	-.10144504***	-.10061856***	-.10121411***	-.10116903***
occupation_8	-.01019046	-.00971794	-.0104076	-.01010831
occupation_9	-.12541047***	-.12508277***	-.12513555***	-.12552281***
round_10	.0042041	.00258998	.00310756	.00281578
round_11	-.00524675	-.00687934	-.00644211	-.0065833
round_12	-.00674471	-.0082841	-.00784437	-.00816691
cheart	-.01282462	-.0135959	-.0118314	-.01302344
clungs	.03941723***	.03918327***	.04054747***	.03694418***
cliver	.01767289*	.01477509	.01618572	.01378418
ckidny	.0009254	.00122756	.00160304	.00111697
cgi	-.00062025	-.00079791	-.00106807	-.00058534
cspine	-.00464508	-.00489828	-.00504277	-.00521482
cother	-.00086547	-.00073189	-.00019993	-.00135145
diabetes_b20	-.03719927			
heart_b20	–			
stroke_b20	-.03803866			
tbc_b20	-.01698457			
hepatitis_b20	-.02917758**			
diabetes_20		-.02750776		
heart_20		.05839574		
stroke_20		.24507382*		
tbc_20		.01060056		
hepatitis_20		.00925964		
diabetes_10			-.04903766	
heart_10			-.01289033	
stroke_10			-.03361457	
tbc_10			-.11833582	
hepatitis_10			-.02558451	
diabetes_5				.02017598
heart_5				.00539258
stroke_5				-.01842532
tbc_5				.19298307***
hepatitis_5				.01203015
constant	4.8475018***	4.8493382***	4.8524877***	4.8500274***
R2	.14135195	.14153691	.14132912	.14158014
N	12009	12009	12009	12009

Notes: * p<.1; ** p<.05; *** p<.01.

Table A.5 RLMS IV regression results – dependent variables: log deflated wage rate (2000 prices) and log weekly worked hours (using self-reported health)

Variable	WRfullsample	WRmale	WRfemale	LSfullsample	LSmale	LSfemale
healthGOOD	.20261634***	.1806543**	.22419709***	-.01000299	.02130741	-.02027266
Gender	.27585464***			.1101072***		
Age	.03614345***	.02352038***	.04389459***	.01683673***	.01700254***	.01448804***
age2	-.00043666***	-.00030836***	-.00051943***	-.00020515***	-.00020695***	-.00017566***
Highsc	.07089832***	.07871912***	.04943325*	-.01161474	-.01891072**	-.00217997
Tecdp	.08644842***	.10692356***	.06991908***	.0033794	-.01350005	.01435595*
Insdp	.31426173***	.2392171***	.34637742***	.00540103	.02079802*	-.00123836
Gradp	-.08415951	-.04194061	-.10088591	.01388915	-.02216501	.04175885
Married	.05141418***	.15022216***	.01163241	-.02538585***	.01937082*	-.03886909***
Tenure	-.00081092	-.00546021*	.00218432	-.00211222**	-.00426801***	-.00063797
tenure2	.00009809	.00019499**	.0000289	-.00005859***	.00011212***	.00001423
Pjemps	8.804e-06***	7.632e-06***	9.004e-06***	-8.013e-07	-9.378e-07	-2.854e-07
Ncat	-.04521146***	.00215761	-.10828932***	.0057746	.01806025**	-.02033957*
Private	.17277442***	.09955215***	.24806507***	.07645701***	.06493953***	.07887115***
region_2	-.0133603	.09148693*	-.0958643**	.05869207***	.06096713***	.05765205***
region_3	-.44289043***	-.40460824***	-.48610782***	.01849206*	.01404615	.01895777
region_4	-.70229557***	-.66428493***	-.7348911***	.03537858***	.01953694	.04064509***
region_5	-.61434647***	-.53340948***	-.67970519***	.07870559***	.05313381***	.09620142***
region_6	-.45873715***	-.33987848***	-.55962049***	.01230895	-.01643169	.03275026**
region_7	-.46645139***	-.45783094***	-.47691641***	.04152007***	.08148437***	.00841795
region_8	-.2853641***	-.2289622***	-.32352706***	.0502703***	.06153782***	.03448115**
Urban	.43761558***	.62312852***	.2831659***	.02274333***	-.01505292*	.04760405***
Occupation_2	-.01146613	-.01094595	-.00256181	-.17491303***	-.1825607***	-.17610764***
Occupation_3	-.09973417***	-.04334927	-.10912741***	-.07085586***	-.0616262***	-.07649988***
Occupation_4	-.15451163***	-.03652103	-.16638103***	-.06779682***	-.05827246*	-.06896023***
Occupation_5	-.41975459***	-.31318111***	-.48718413***	.08981792***	.0592768***	.10308978***
Occupation_6	-.47198821***	-.37263434***	-.84237456***	-.028839<8	-.04008518	-.03736733
Occupation_7	-.03552898	-.05105415	-.05908826	-.10097471***	-.10827515***	-.02649565
Occupation_8	-.10721544***	-.12569034***	-.04693364	-.01031805	-.01859227	.00006369
Occupation_9	-.48071172***	-.55627943***	-.42828469***	-.12501984***	-.0406391**	-.18950645***
round_10	.17584632***	.20261341***	.15252564***	.00302858	-.0035675	.00816274
round_11	.37643375***	.35788906***	.39169577***	-.00642209	-.00452699	-.00850983
round_12	.46681949***	.49302316***	.44638437***	-.00806678	-.01231146	-.00638784
Constant	1.0524022***	1.3785507***	1.0700368***	4.857801<***	4.9607769***	4.8823367***
R2	.38005142	.37336365	.37954554	.14009513	.10294687	.13476493
N	11297	5081	6216	12009	5425	6584
Sargan	13.573047	11.927898	12.401589	17.049472	13.678117	19.081833
sargan p	.25752479	.36908726	.33422615	.10642072	.25131896	.0596403

Notes: * p<.1; ** p<.05; *** p<.01; health measure: self-reported health status.

Table A.6 RLMS IV regression results – dependent variables: log deflated wage rate (2000 prices) and log weekly worked hours (using work-days missed owing to illness)

Variable	WRfullsample	WRmale	WRfemale	LSfullsample	LSmale	LSfemale
Misseddays	-.05380539***	-.03690035*	-.05546552***	.00321319	-.00709594	.01402738*
Gender	.29772264***			.10998022***		
Age	.03114485***	.01850996***	.04046707***	.01721108***	.01632242***	.0147364***
age2	-.00040003***	-.00026616***	-.00050769***	-.00020857***	-.00020076***	-.00017564***
Highsc	.0764457***	.08810853***	.04997693*	-.01159807	-.01808313*	-.00146113
Tecdp	.08665504***	.1073604***	.06226547***	.0031956	-.01300065	.01608852*
Insdp	.31530499***	.24677968***	.33882159***	.00571132	.02204791*	.00141949
Gradp	-.0787445	-.036784	-.08761471	.01393563	-.02159379	.04096062
Married	.05356679***	.15083713***	.01173622	-.02579732***	.01930354*	-.03936297***
Tenure	-.00122834	-.00524941	.00082434	-.00211588**	-.00420651***	-.00045703
tenure2	.00011241*	.00019362**	.00006644	-.0005821**	.00011106***	8.823e-06
Pjemps	9.280e-06***	8.407e-06***	8.816e-06***	-8.50e-07	-8.565e-07	-3.074e-07
Ncat	-.04023962***	.00362648	-.09662369***	.000693	.01770139***	-.02175956***
Private	.16724902***	.09387912***	.24856076***	.07756117***	.06402571***	.08025452***
region_2	-.01474598	.09875703***	-.11009453***	.0577796***	.06201305***	.057782***
region_3	-.4558448***	-.42070126***	-.49921143***	.01890107*	.01165807	.01929232
region_4	-.71430958***	-.66690059***	-.75631568***	.03665627***	.01863438	.04386867***
region_5	-.61081329***	-.5267249***	-.68255719***	.07879792***	.05402857***	.09821436***
region_6	-.47894979***	-.34875802***	-.59416784***	.01363934	-.0175098	.03771347***
region_7	-.48772765***	-.46787374***	-.5126407***	.04312625***	.08002961***	.01396134
region_8	-.29416799***	-.23611033***	-.33333955***	.05040509***	.06036483***	.03431264**
Urban	.44175078***	.62699818***	.28495936***	.02193919***	-.01431369	.04659559***
Occupation_2	-.027564	-.04925416	-.0844466	-.17300785***	-.18745121***	-.1760129***
Occupation_3	-.12230053***	-.05608059	-.1344305***	-.06794825***	-.06362624***	-.07169013***
Occupation_4	-.17091698***	-.0763228	-.18042962***	-.06618904***	-.06534309**	-.0677314***
Occupation_5	-.43565594***	-.2985637***	-.52124317***	.09266941***	.06085781***	.11050034***
Occupation_6	-.48343043***	-.38829406***	-.7552105***	-.02690202	-.04387496	-.05866459
Occupation_7	-.04122031	-.05320954	-.07698807	-.10081479***	-.10856194***	-.02472499
Occupation_8	-.12073531***	-.13498605***	-.0576109	-.00918769	-.01997502	.00046696
Occupation_9	-.50227005***	-.56088127***	-.46485105***	-.12261359***	-.04186336**	-.18370621***
round_10	.17884361***	.20508534***	.15430605***	.00259199	-.0038077	.00628939
round_11	.38042079***	.36002555***	.39748229***	-.00650397	-.00496189	-.00990774
round_12	.46644317***	.49288934***	.44663449***	-.00755301	-.01312552	-.0643482
Constant	1.3008961***	1.6037212***	1.3262024***	4.8369351***	4.9923983***	4.8495011***
R2	.32233376	.34607243	.31337964	.13220628	.09785919	.11655025
N	11 297	5 081	6 216	12 009	5 425	6 584
Sargan	10.582327	13.854043	8.4962567	15.267294	13.358761	15.893294
sargan p	.47888791	.24117537	.66828023	.17058417	.27052497	.14513876

Notes: * p<.1; ** p<.05; *** p<.01; health measure: missed days due to ill-health.

Table A.7 *NOBUS IV regression results – dependent variable: log monthly wage rate*

Variable	Full	Male	Female
healthGOOD	.23073613***	.29161317***	.18554934***
Age	.00194805	.00285506	.00034706
Male	.2827457***		
Children	-.0186142	.01235114	-.05409407***
Private	.04593329**	-.02217283	.16266443***
schooling2	.17295232***	.18103981***	.14660409***
schooling3	.42042849***	.40874823***	.44509322***
experience 2	.15488742***	.21468458***	.09025464**
experience 3	.27605528***	.33826986***	.19469783***
experience 4	.29482454***	.3339668***	.24849332***
experience 5	.30288889***	.28737294***	.36047057***
		[98 omitted regional dummies]	
Urban	.36058887***	.45050028***	.20029591***
Constant	6.3669247***	6.468474***	6.7210779***
R2	.35884352	.34130484	.41305857
N	4 139	2 410	1 729
Sargan	2.3231368	4.2421652	.15670567
sargan p	.12746276	.03943185	.69220781

Notes: * p<.1; ** p<.05; *** p<.01; healthGOOD instrumented by father and mother health status.
Source: NOBUS Dataset round 1: sample of jobholders whose family includes the parents.

Table A.8 *NOBUS IV regression results – dependent variable: log weekly worked hours*

Variable	Full	Male	Female
healthGOOD	.03167153	.03403846	.02639951
Age	.00021789	-.00028859	.00090962
Male	.04823373***		
Children	.01161265**	.01740233**	.00588029
Private	.04238258***	.02611874**	.06846073***
schooling 2	-.00202497	-.00121966	.0023968
schooling 3	-.0291298***	-.02807691*	-.02598168
experience 2	.02950427**	.03812825**	.01756524
experience 3	.04732545***	.05443608***	.04033184*
experience 4	.04869325***	.06112273***	.03543496
experience 5	.04743424**	.0745132***	.01398805
		[98 omitted regional dummies]	
Urban	.00093956	-.01060702	.02084233
Constant	3.4491043***	3.4881173***	3.460679***
R2	.0451653	.04935113	.07885763
N	4 488	2 655	1 833
Sargan	2.9013272	1.909446	.56854037
sargan p	.08850665	.16702481	.45083952

Notes: * p<.1; ** p<.05; *** p<.01; healthGOOD instrumented by father and mother health status.
Source: NOBUS Dataset round 1: Sample of jobholders whose family includes the parents.

Panel regressions

Table A.9 PANEL – dependent variable: log deflated wage rate (2000 prices): males

Variable	OLS	RE	FE	HT	AM
Age	.02117373*	.03060971*	.03371538	.01813034	.0234186
age2	-.02543067**	-.03546528*	-.02382196	-.0311323	-.0213325
Tenure	-.00772551	-.01517426**	-.0206151***	-.01909465**	-.01806072***
tenure2	.01210427	.04237933**	.06945062***	.06422693***	.0584895***
P;emps	9.530e-06***	9.788e-06**	9.429e-06	.0000118**	.00001127**
Private	.04570286	.03499996	.03313663	.0309431	.02631349
Married	.14033812**	-.03676585	-.22294367**	-.20775497**	-.15196781*
Ncat	-.05326126	-.01793909	.00538132	.01683112	-.00097233
healthGOOD	.13197755***	.09158229***	.07569402*	.07786367**	.0755662**
Occupation_2	-.01218971	.00225306	.0043603	.00617929	.0022-176
Occupation_3	-.05167111	.02008562	.05246994	.05219877	.05232641
occupation_4	-.19906217	.2181705	.39427491**	.39282628***	.37307211**
occupation_5	-.24020772**	-.02854871	.125755	.13997179	.11371703
occupation_6	-.94112994**	-.17614337	.10702769	.10056151	.0679691
occupation_7	.0386432	.10132112	.12744936	.12405609	.11974571
occupation_8	-.0429258	.00489442	.03180318	.03342481	.02176699
occupation_9	-.57218885***	-.28322658***	-.07798007	-.07972034	-.10124062
region_2	.27892274**	.29314799	—	.25565869	.26318595
region_3	-.29012799***	-.2835072*	—	-.41834883	-.32384047
region_4	-.48320866***	-.50339542***	—	-.62553843**	-.56938138**
region_5	-.39498039***	-.40471495*	—	-.37981395	-.37930179
region_6	-.13100975	-.13158781	—	-.26354191	-.16251081
region_7	-.65294516***	-.67053312***	—	-.70585965**	-.72745543***
region_8	-.08770838	-.05826851	—	-.12961441	-.09358942
urban	.53909976***	.52193122***	—	.32506656	.39969081***
round_10	.168135***	.16313149***	.14594161***	.15260468***	.15493627**
round_11	.38907013***	.37849082***	.34758368***	.36074622***	.36456176***
round_12	.49593055***	.485547***	.44142583***	.46017735***	.46584738***
school_1	.25757494***	.32212736***	—	.81691085	.83514246**
school_2	.40336141***	.49213283***	—	1.9765633**	1.2196359***
school_3	.63699184***	.7444805***	—	1.4499061	1.3256559***
school_4	.66247112***	.72739066***	—	.17519122	.57196294
constant	1.160447***	1.0129677***	1.3497267	.74809819	.74063887
N	1096	1096	1096	1096	1096

Notes: * p<.1; ** p<.05; *** p<.01; Hausman test fixed effects vs random effect: chi2(20) = 40.65; Prob>chi2 = 0.0041; Hausman test fixed effects vs Hausman-Taylor: chi2(19) = 1.12; Prob>chi2 = 1.0000; Hausman test Hausman-Taylor vs Amemiya-Macurdy: chi2(19) = 3.08; Prob>chi2 = 1.0000; FE: fixed effects; OLS: ordinary least squares; RE: random effects; HT: Hausman-Taylor; AM: Amemiya-Macurdy.

Table A.10 *PANEL – dependent variable: log weekly worked hours: males*

Variable	OLS	RE	FE	HT	AM
Age	.00968936**	.01011673	.014124	.00773793	.00550749
age2	-.01130532**	-.01229069*	-.0820846	-.01072686	-.0061599
Tenure	-.00395814*	-.00350348	-.0269069	-.0029343	-.00371731
tenure2	.01254271*	.01316617	.1322701	.01425271*	.0161937*
Pjemps	-1.109e-06	-5.444e-07	1.23e-06	2.967e-07	-1.640e-07
Private	.05022197***	.02641639	-.0345284	.00441571	.00623633
Married	.09359559***	.07396736*	.4708204	.04284235	.05958309
Ncat	.01429715	.02212276	.2753488	.02416649	.03011741
healthGOOD	-.01965858	-.01468967	-.137866	-.01445042	-.0149034
Occupation_2	-.21092642***	-.12738774***	-.4395166	-.0441609	-.04812057
Occupation_3	-.1103376***	-.1005106***	-.0634389***	-.09603576***	-.0996362***
Occupation_4	-.0852414	-.17208368***	-.0984353***	-.20838166***	-.20470985***
Occupation_5	.03435495	.02383147	-.1944352	.0153265	.01634753
Occupation_6	-.00552382	-.04861333	-.707335	-.06588934	-.05051898
Occupation_7	-.17901824***	-.1455056***	-.1574215***	-.11468832***	-.11785297***
Occupation_8	-.09831434***	-.08156896**	-.5571441	-.06633536	-.0683112
Occupation_9	-.03111297	-.01936531	-.1017347	-.00940763	-.00781331
region_2	.07384698	.07319388	—	.09981761	.06052615
region_3	-.0642961*	-.06370392	—	-.07252672	-.07501232
region_4	-.07546378*	-.07729309	—	-.10336157	-.0865404
region_5	-.03169123	-.02565908	—	.03149358	-.04685389
region_6	-.08640749**	-.08861418	—	-.08514215	-.11174203
region_7	-.0443195	-.04286526	—	-.04661855	-.03856058
region_8	-.06315885	-.07427061	—	-.11929904	-.07699556
Urban	-.01937896	-.01609842	—	-.07301517	-.01544788
round_10	.00777308	.01059797	.816888	.0139167	.01233232
round_11	-.00697861	-.00330935	.917258	.00074844	-.00239133
round_12	-.00645034	-.00263858	.457219	.00227273	-.00210441
school_1	-.05903512**	-.0635665	—	.12727169	-.14966983
school_2	-.08106482***	-.08653917*	—	.22689688	-.03809073
school_3	-.05420356	-.0688878	—	.3848647	-.24634658
school_4	-.07648919	-.14565492	—	.39316961	-.92683147
Constant	5.2020154***	5.1969917***	5.382847***	5.0510247***	5.3499498***
N	1096	1096	1096	1096	1096

Notes: * p<.1; ** p<.05; *** p<.01; Hausman test fixed effects vs random effect: chi2(20)= 28.21; Prob>chi2 = 0.1 -46; Hausman test fixed effects vs Hausman–Taylor: chi2(19)= 0.55; Prob>chi2 = 1.0000; Hausman test Hausman–Taylor vs Amemiya-Macurdy: chi2(19) = 1.71; Prob>chi2 = 1.0000; OLS: ordinary least squares; RE: random effects; FE: fixed effects; HT: Hausman–Taylor; AM: Amemiya-Macurdy.

Table A.11 PANEL – dependent variable: log deflated wage ʿrate (2000 prices): females

Variable	OLS	RE	FE	HT	AM
Age	.04884346***	.06736967***	.10066973***	.10790077***	.10325259***
age2	-.05421362***	-.07580477***	-.15605471***	-.15072374***	-.13079675***
tenure	-.00005831	-.00346258	-.00820986	-.00729327	-.00662808
tenure2	-.00103402	.00719763	.02147504	.01986644	.01643053
pjemps	.00001359***	.00001239***	-5.603e-06	1.181e-06	1.233e-06
private	.22376717***	.072317**	-.01437716	-.0136186	-.01310365
married	.00028125	.00738042	.01341194	.01071813	.01188477
ncat	-.10801699***	-.07377408**	-.04957205	-.05391545	-.05380167
healthGOOD	.00899523	.03121741	.02602269	.02761743	.02923847
occupation_2	.05577093	.07850739	.06758284	.06643888	.06439402
occupation_3	-.0153171	.02146124	.03148909	.03083616	.03104208
occupation_4	-.11040535*	-.06521419	-.04835037	-.04741679	-.04775724
occupation_5	-.54344458***	-.2801505***	.01557992	.02031464	.01952723
occupation_7	.08008339	.06526647	.00884341	.01068766	.01395186
occupation_8	-.05201295	-.03782227	-.07510576	-.06741964	-.0661714
occupation_9	-.45957353***	-.20444463**	.09278365	.09481375	.09614351
region_2	-.13999192*	-.20911144		-.48590165	-.34880907
region_3	-.50231503***	-.53116243***		-.45795033	-.53031251
region_4	-.74096226***	-.77493104***		-.89981922**	-.8733(?)9**
region_5	-.63540426***	-.69525462***		-.6915516	-.78563166*
region_6	-.5473698***	-.57912027***		-.78280566	-.71864947*
region_7	-.62834388***	-.66565366***		-.90982369	-.80104975*
region_8	-.37340449***	-.43559004***		-.56746261	-.56762899
urban	.15423442***	.18812914***		.36136134	.25022075
round_10	.18149427***	.1928466(?)***	.2380016***	.22420629***	.21243407***
round_11	.45971719***	.4719790(?)***	.55111916***	.52550048***	.50231554***
round_12	.51680043***	.5310405(?)***	.64696711***	.60956004***	.5742841***
school_1	.1944843**	.1891697(?)		-6.0365962	-1.5936188
school_2	.25540653*	.3006058(?)*		-6.093138	-1.2300934
school_3	.57598761***	.6274978***		-4.4909463	-.75936396
school_4	.681436***	.74557585***		-.8708852	1.1328886
Constant	.84034209***	.4156382(?)	.38980734	5.8148068	1.4537398
N	1904	1904	1904	1904	1904

Notes: * p<.1; ** p<.05; *** p<.01; Hausman test fixed effects vs random effect: chi2(20) = 64.56; Prob>chi2 = 0.0000; Hausman test fixed effects vs Hausman-Taylor: chi2(19) = 2.23; Prob>chi2 = 1.0000; Hausman test Hausman-Taylor vs Amemiya-Macurdy: chi2(19) = 2.39; Prob>chi2 = 1.0000; OLS: ordinary least squares; RE: random effects; FE: fixed effects; HT: Hausman-Taylor; AM: Amemiya-Macurdy.

Table A.12 *PANEL – dependent variable: log weekly worked hours: females*

Variable	OLS	RE	FE	HT	AM
Age	.01405474***	.00713686	-.22876607***	-.02768314**	-.02504998**
age2	-.01520261***	-.00682048	.24564225***	.04468031***	.03637539***
tenure	.00018417	.0015545	.00491668*	.0046434*	.00428144*
tenure2	-.00177468	-.00700912	-.01839697***	-.01760554*	-.0160395**
pjemps	-7.685e-07	-2.912e-07	-2.333e-06	-2.617e-06	-2.063e-06
private	.0723087***	.02815004*	-.0652035	-.00634699	-.00584964
married	-.06523011***	-.05414285***	-.01885375	-.01718639	-.02338578
ncat	-.04694642***	-.05493409***	-.06310345***	-.0632857***	-.06176603***
healthGOOD	-.01529577	-.02104664	-.2394817	-.02400828	-.0243819*
occupation_2	-.13872762***	-.07864605***	-.21027135	-.01049274	-.01060721
occupation_3	-.04832293***	-.02975507	-.22232382	-.02192721	-.02245031
occupation_4	.00178738	.01370745	-.21396924	-.01365074	-.01291123
occupation_5	.20324933***	.1690263***	.24756556	.04767363	.04907036
occupation_7	.00249755	.02887341	.2006936	.01969135	.01862799
occupation_8	.06178278**	.07571579**	.622016	.06197632	.06119144
occupation_9	-.06500797**	-.05805535	-.191641**	-.11816436**	-.11771333***
region_2	.04269644	.03478438	—	.14238722	.06589317
region_3	.00976103	.00053723	—	-.01808684	-.00896455
region_4	.05898428**	.05603467	—	.24275572	.09263906
region_5	.08703557***	.07217828	—	.19255138	.0737897
region_6	.01526735	.00665344	—	.26225193	.07547088
region_7	-.02668769	-.02780075	—	.2432143	.03633142
region_8	.0230401	.02041398	—	.21246341	.07272393
urban	.06394156***	.06786983***	-.0893178	.01321326	.07288475
round_10	-.00400421	-.00251684	-.1726122	-.00912039	-.004995
round_11	-.0074286	-.00476587	-.406428*	-.01767266	-.00950599
round_12	-.01834118	-.01732908	—	-.04128489*	-.0286993*
school_1	.21837139***	.20248681***	—	5.6885155	.99684116
school_2	.2593469***	.23333548***	—	4.8112981*	.91200172
school_3	.2436505***	.194317***	—	5.1919824	.7156517
school_4	.298923***	.23065273**	—	2.1060542	-.56722012
constant	4.6019202***	4.7393288***	5.207691***	.27965245	4.5953589***
N	1904	1904	1904	1904	1904

Notes: * p<.1; ** p<.05; *** p<.01; Hausman test fixed effects vs random effect: chi2(20) = 59.37; Prob>chi2 = 0.000; Hausman test fixed effects vs Hausman-Taylor: chi2(19) = 0.60; Prob>chi2 = 1.0000; Hausman test Hausman-Taylor vs Anemiya-Macurdy: chi2(19) = 2.47; Prob>chi2 = 1.0000; OLS: ordinary least squares; RE: random effects; FE: fixed effects; HT: Hausman-Taylor; AM: Anemiya-Macurdy.

References

Alsan, M, Bloom, DE and Canning, D (2004). *The effect of population health on foreign direct investment.* NBER Working Paper 10596. Cambridge, MA, National Bureau of Economic Research.

Amemiya, T and Macurdy, TE (1986). Instrumental-variable estimation of an error components model. *Econometrica*, 54: 869–881.

Andreev, EM et al. (2003). The evolving pattern of avoidable mortality in Russia. *International Journal of Epidemiology*, 32: 437–446.

Andreev, EM, McKee, M and Shkolnikov, V (2003). Health expectancy in the Russian Federation: a new perspective on the health divide in Europe. *Bulletin of the World Health Organization*, 1(11): 778–787.

Balabanova, D, Falkingham, J and McKee, M (2003). Winners and losers: the expansion of insurance coverage in Russia in the 1990s. *American Journal of Public Health*, 93: 2124–2130.

Baldwin, M, Zeager, L and Flacco, P (1994). Gender differences in wage losses from impairments. *Journal of Human Resources*, 29: 865–887.

Barro, R (1996). *Health and economic growth.* Washington, DC, Pan American Health Organization (PAHO) Program on Public Policy and Health.

Barro, R (1997). *Determinants of economic growth: a cross-country empirical study.* Cambridge, MA, MIT Press.

Bartel, A and Taubman, P (1979). Health and labor market success: the role of various diseases. *The Review of Economics and Statistics*, 61(1): 1–8.

Berkovec, J and Stern, S (1991). Job exit behavior of older men. *Econometrica*, 59: 189–210.

Bhargava, A, Jamison, DT and Murray, C (2001). Modelling the effects of health on economic growth. *Journal of Health Economics*, 20: 423–440.

Bloom, D, Canning, D and Sevilla, J (2001). *The effect of health on economic growth: theory and evidence.* NBER Working Paper 8587. Cambridge, MA, National Bureau of Economic Research.

Bloom, D, Canning, D and Sevilla, J (2002). *Health, worker productivity and economic growth.* Pittsburgh, School of Public Policy and Management, Carnegie Mellon University.

Bloom, DE, Canning, D and Graham, B (2003). Longevity and life-cycle savings. *Scandinavian Journal of Economics*, 105: 319–338.

Bloom, DE, Canning, D and Jamison, DT (2004). Health, wealth and welfare. *Finance and development*, 41(1): 10–15.

Bobak, M et al. (2006). Changes in smoking prevalence in Russia, 1996–2004. *Tobacco Control*, 15: 131–135.

Bound, J, Stinebrickner, T and Waidmann, T (2003). *Health, economic resources and the work decisions of older men*. Bethesda, MD, Canadian National Institute on Aging.

Cercone, JA (1994). *Alcohol-related problems as an obstacle to the development of human capital*. World Bank Technical Paper No. 219. Washington, DC, World Bank.

CMH (2001). *Macroeconomics and health: investing in health for economic development*. Report of the Commission on Macroeconomics and Health. Geneva, World Health Organization.

Coile, C (2003). *Health shocks and couples' labor supply decisions*. CRR Working Paper No. 08. Boston, MA, Center for Retirement Research (Boston College).

Costa, D and Kahn, M (2004). Changes in the value of life: 1940–1980. *Journal of Risk and Uncertainty*, 29(2): 159–180.

Cotoyannis, P and Rice, N (2001). The impact of health on wages: evidence from the British Household Panel Survey. *Empirical Economics*, 26: 599–622.

Crafts, N (2003). *The contribution of increased life expectancy to growth of living standards in the UK, 1870–2001*. [Unpublished manuscript]. London, London School of Economics and Political Science.

Currie, J and Madrian, BC (1999). Health, health insurance and the labor market. In: Ashenfelter, O and Card, D (eds). *Handbook of Labor Economics*, 3(50): 3309–3416.

Cutler, D and Richardson, E (1997). Measuring the health of the US population. *Brookings Papers on Economic Activity: Microeconomics*, Vol 1997: 217–271.

Davis, C (2005). *Economic consequences of changes in the health status of the population and economic benefits of medical programmes in the USSR during 1950–1991*. Background paper prepared for the forthcoming report on health and economic development in eastern Europe and central Asia. Copenhagen, WHO Regional Office for Europe.

European Foundation for the Improvement of Living and Working Conditions (1997). *Preventing absenteeism at the workplace*. Luxembourg, European Foundation for the Improvement of Living and Working Conditions.

European Foundation for the Improvement of Living and Working Conditions (2001). *Third European Working Conditions Survey (2000)*. Dublin, European Foundation for the Improvement of Living and Working Conditions.

Gallup, JL and Sachs, JD, with Andrew Mellinger (1999). *Geography and economic development*. CID Working Paper No. 1. Cambridge, MA, Center for International Development.

Hausman, JA (1978). Specification tests in econometrics. *Econometrica*, 46: 1251–1271.

Hausman, JA and Taylor, WE (1981). Panel data and unobservable individual effects. *Econometrica*, 49: 1377–1398.

Haveman, R et al. (1994). Market work, wages and men's health. *Journal of Health Economics*, 13: 163–182.

Heckman, J, Ichimura, H and Todd, P (1997). Matching as an econometric evaluation estimator: evidence from evaluating a job training programme. *Review of Economic Studies*, 64: 605–654.

Islam, N (1995). Growth empirics: a panel data approach. *Quarterly Journal of Economics*, 110(4): 1127–1170.

Jamison, D, Lau, L and Wang, J (2004). *Health's contribution to economic growth in an environment of partially endogenous technical progress.* Disease Control Priorities Project Working Paper 10. Bethesda, MD, Fogarty International Centre, National Institutes of Health.

Jiménez-Martín, S, Labeaga, JM and Martínez, M (1999). *Health status and retirement decisions for older European couples.* Brussels, European Commission TMR Programme.

Kalemli-Ozcan, S, Ryder, HE and Weil, DN (2000). Mortality decline, human capital investment and economic growth. *Journal of Development Economics*, 62: 1–23.

Ladnaia, N, Pokrovsky, V and Rühl, C (2003). *The economic consequences of HIV in Russia: an interactive simulation approach.* Moscow, World Bank.

Levine, R and Renelt, D (1992). A sensitivity analysis of cross-country growth regressions. *American Economic Review*, 82: 942–963.

Lock, K et al. (2002). The health impact of the International Development Targets on life expectancy in the Russian Federation. *Journal of Health Policy and Planning*, 17(3): 257–263.

McKee, M et al. (2005). The composition of surrogate alcohols consumed in Russia. *Alcohol Clinical and Experimental Research*, 29: 1884–1888.

McMichael, AJ et al. (2004). Mortality trends and setbacks: global convergence or divergence? *Lancet*, 363: 1155–1159.

Miller, TR (2000). Variations between countries in values of statistical life. *Journal of Transport Economics and Policy*, 34(2): 169–188.

Mitchell, J and Burkhauser, R (1990). Disentangling the effect of arthritis on earnings: a simultaneous estimate of wage rates and hours worked. *Applied Economics Letters*, 22: 1291–1310.

Mullahy, J (1991). Gender differences in labor market effects of alcoholism. *American Economic Review* (Papers and Proceedings), 81(2): 161–165.

Nickel, S (1981). Biases in dynamic models with fixed effects. *Econometrica*, 49: 1117–1126.

Nolte, E, McKee, M and Gilmore, A (2005). Morbidity and mortality in transition countries in the European context. In: Macura, M, MacDonald, A and Haug, W. (eds). *The new demographic regime: population challenges and policy responses.* New York and Geneva, United Nations: 153–176.

Nordhaus, W (2003). The health of nations: the contribution of improved health to living standards. In: Moss, M (ed.). *The measurement of economic and social performance.* New York, Columbia University Press for the National Bureau of Economic Research: 193–226.

Pauly, M et al. (2002). A general model of the impact of absenteeism on employers and employees. *Health Economics*, 11: 221–231.

Pelkowski, JM and Berger, MC (2004). The impact of health on employment, wages and hours worked over the life cycle. *Quarterly Review of Economics and Finance*, 44: 102–121.

Rechel, B, Shapo, L and McKee, M (2004). *Millennium Development Goals for health in Europe and Central Asia.* Washington, DC, World Bank.

Rese, A et al. (2005). Implementing general practice in Russia: getting beyond the first steps. *British Medical Journal*, 331: 204–207.

Rivera, B and Currais, L (1999). Economic growth and health: direct impact or reverse causation? *Applied Economics Letters*, 6: 761–764.

Rosembaum, P, and Rubin, D (1983). The central role of the propensity score in observational studies for causal effects. *Biometrika*, 70: 41–55.

Sachs, J and Warner, A (1995). Economic reform and the process of global integration. *Brookings Papers on Economic Activity*, Vol. 1995: 1–118.

Sala-I-Martin, X, Doppelhofer, G and Miller, RI (2004). Determinants of long-term growth: a Bayesian Averaging of Classical Estimates (BACE) approach. *American Economic Review*, 94(4): 813–835.

Sammartino, FJ (1987). The effect of health on retirement. *Social Security Bulletin*, 50(2): 31–47.

Sargan, JD (1958). The estimation of economic relationships using instrumental variables. *Econometrica*, 26: 397–415.

Schultz, TP and Tansel, A (1995). *Measurement of returns to adult health: morbidity effects on wage rates in Cote d'Ivoire and Ghana.* Living Standards Measurement Study Working Paper No. 95. Washington, DC, World Bank.

Shkolnikov, V, McKee, M and Leon, DA (2001). Changes in life expectancy in Russia in the mid-1990s, *Lancet*, 357: 917–921.

Shkolnikov, V et al. (2004). Mortality reversal in Russia: the story so far. *Hygeia Internationalis*, 4: 29–80.

Siddiqui, S (1997). The impact of health on retirement behaviour: empirical evidence from West Germany. *Econometrics and Health Economics*, 6: 425–438.

Stern, S (1989). Measuring the effect of disability on labor force participation. *Journal of Human Resources*, 24(3): 361–395.

Stern, S (1996). Measuring child work and residence adjustments to parents' long-term care needs. *Gerontologist*, 36: 76–87.

Strauss, J and Thomas, D (1998). Health, nutrition and economic development. *Journal of Economic Literature*, 36: 766–777.

Suhrcke, M et al. (2005). *The contribution of health to the economy in the European Union.* Brussels, European Commission.

Sullivan, DF (1971). A single index of mortality and morbidity. *Health Services and Mental Health Administration (HSMHA) Health Reports*, 86: 347–354.

Thomas, D (2001). *Health, nutrition and economic prosperity: a microeconomic perspective.* CMH Working Paper No. WG1:7. Geneva, World Health Organization Commission on Macroeconomics and Health.

Tragakes, E and Lessof, S (2003). *Health care systems in transition: Russian Federation.* Brussels, European Observatory on Health Systems and Policies.

Trognon, A (1978). Miscellaneous asymptotic properties of ordinary least squares and maximum likelihood estimators in dynamic error components models. *Annales de l'INSEE*, 30/31: 631–657.

Usher, D (1973). An imputation to the measure of economic growth for changes in life expectancy. In: Moss, M (ed). *The measurement of economic and social performance.* New York, Columbia University Press for National Bureau of Economic Research: 193–226.

Viscusi, WK and Aldy, JE (2003). *The value of statistical life: a critical review of market estimates throughout the world.* NBER Working Paper No. 9487. Cambridge, MA, National Bureau of Economic Research.

WHO (2005). WHO Mortality Database [online database]. Geneva, World Health Organization (http://www3.who.int/whosis/, accessed 1 October 2006).

WHO Regional Office for Europe (2006). European Health for All database (HFA-DB) [online database]. Copenhagen, WHO Regional Office for Europe (http://www.euro.who.int/hfadb, accessed 1 July 2006).

World Bank (2003). *World development indicators, 2003.* Washington, DC, World Bank.

World Bank (2004). *World development indicators, 2004.* Washington, DC, World Bank.

World Bank (2005). *Dying too young: addressing premature mortality and ill health due to noncommunicable diseases and injuries in the Russian Federation (2005).* Washington, DC, World Bank.

Yach, D and Hawkes, C (2004). *The WHO long-term strategy for prevention and control of leading chronic diseases* [draft] (February). Geneva, World Health Organization.

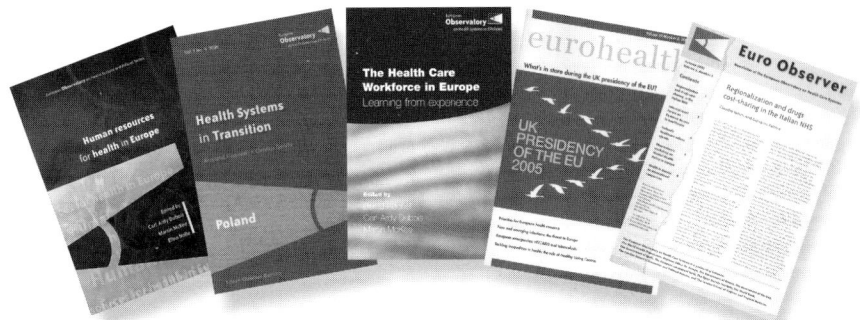

*The European Observatory on Health Systems and Policies
produces a wide range of analytical work on health systems and policies.
Its publishing programme includes:*

☐ **The Health Systems in Transition profiles (HiTs).** Country-based reports that provide a detailed description of the health systems of European and selected OECD countries outside the region, and of policy initiatives in progress or under development.

HiT profiles are downloadable from: www.euro.who.int/observatory

☐ **Joint Observatory/Open University Press/McGraw-Hill Series. A prestigious health series exploring key issues for health systems and policies in Europe.**
Titles include: Mental Health Policy and Practice across Europe ■ Decentralization in Health Care ■ Primary Care in the Driver's Seat ■ Human Resources for Health in Europe ■ Purchasing to Improve Health Systems Performance ■ Social Health Insurance Systems in Western Europe ■ Regulating Pharmaceuticals in Europe

Copies of the books can be ordered from: www.mcgraw-hill.co.uk

☐ **The Occasional Studies.** A selection of concise volumes, presenting evidence-based information on crucial aspects of health, health systems and policies. Recent titles include: Patient Mobility in the EU ■ Private Medical Insurance in the UK ■ The Health Care Workforce in Europe ■ Making Decisions on Public Health ■ Health Systems Transition: learning from experience

Studies are downloadable from: www.euro.who.int/observatory

☐ **Policy briefs.** A series of compact brochures, highlighting key policy lessons on priority issues for Europe's decision-makers, such as cross-border health care, screening, health technology assessment, care outside the hospital.

Policy briefs are downloadable from: www.euro.who.int/observatory

☐ *Eurohealth.* A joint Observatory/LSE Health journal, providing a platform for policy-makers, academics and politicians to express their views on European health policy.

☐ *Euro Observer.* A health policy bulletin, published quarterly, providing information on key health policy issues and health system reforms across Europe.

✳ ✳ ✳ Join our E-Bulletin ✳ ✳ ✳

Are you interested in signing up for the European Observatory's listserve to receive E-Bulletins on news about health systems, electronic versions of our latest publications, upcoming conferences and other news items? If so, please subscribe by sending a blank e-mail to: subscribe-observatory_listserve@list.euro.who.int